Debra Adelaide is the mother of two children, Joe 'Tex' and Ellen. She has worked as a university teacher and researcher and is now an author, freelance editor, and occasional book reviewer. She is the author or editor/introducer of seven books, and has contributed to several others. Her novel *The Hotel Albatross* appeared in 1994. *Motherlove* was published in 1995.

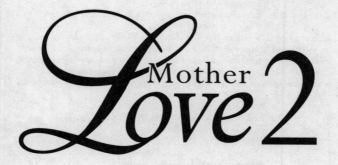

Mother Love 2

More stories about
Births, Babies & Beyond

Edited by Debra Adelaide

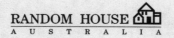

RANDOM HOUSE
AUSTRALIA

Random House Australia Pty Ltd
20 Alfred Street, Milsons Point, NSW 2061
http://www.randomhouse.com.au

Sydney   New York   Toronto
London   Auckland   Johannesburg
and agencies throughout the world

First published in 1997

National Library of Australia
Cataloguing-in-Publication-data:

Motherlove 2: more stories about births, babies and beyond.

ISBN 0 09 183512 7.

1. Love, Maternal–Literary collections. 2. Australian
prose literature–20th century. 3. Australian
prose literature–Women authors. I. Adelaide, Debra, 1958- .
II. Title: Mother love 2.

A828.308080354

Cover photograph by Lesley O'Donnell
Designed by Mary Callahan
Typeset in 11.5,15.5 Goudy by Midland Typesetters, Maryborough
Printed by Griffin Paperbacks, Adelaide

for my sister,
Bronwyn,
and her children,
Harry and Phoebe

Acknowledgements

This book would never have been organised and completed on time without assistance. In this case it was from my dear friend Gabrielle Carey, who steadfastly refused to be talked, bullied, tricked or otherwise persuaded into being my co-editor, but who agreed instead to accept some 'work' from me and to help in return for a mere acknowledgement in the book. For her diligent and cheerful approach to all those phone calls, faxes and letters that kept track of so many of the contributors, Gabrielle has my heartfelt thanks. She also performed miracles with stubborn or secretive discs, enabling me to get on with the task of editing much more efficiently; and, finally, provided her own editorial input, which I greatly appreciated.

Thanks also to my publisher Margaret Sullivan for inviting me to do this volume and for her confidence that it would be as good as the last one.

And a special thanks to all the contributors to *Motherlove 2*: working on this book has been a pleasure and a privilege because of their commitment and generosity of spirit.

Contents

DEBRA ADELAIDE
Introduction 1

JANE CADZOW
Love that Moves the Sun 9

SUE INGLETON
A Letter to Roxane 19

DEBRA OSWALD
Caesarians, Storkmarks and Other People's Children 29

GRETEL KILLEEN
Mouse 43

ROSIE SCOTT
Birth Diaries 55

URSULA DUBOSARSKY
Alone Like a Stone 65

MARGARET SIMONS
Why Clare is Not a Yahoo 77

JILL SINGER
The Shadow Behind Me 99

JENNY TABAKOFF
Bed 109

PENNY BIGGINS
Nature's Quirky Little Ways 121

DEBBIE SPILLANE
One Rung Below an Axe-Murderer 133

FIONA GILES
Two Breasts, Twelve Weeks 151

DONNA MCDONALD
I am a Mother 173

SUSAN JOHNSON
This is My Life 181

KARINA KELLY
Living in Colour 193

TRISHA GODDARD
A Tale of Two Pregnancies 205

LEONIE STEVENS
Mother Superior and the Kid from Hell 221

SALLY MCINERNEY
Field Notes on Sleeping and Waking 239

KERRY CUE
War of the Words 255

CANDIDA BAKER
Just a Little One, Dear 263

ANNE KIRKPATRICK
Travelling Another Road 281

CHRISTINE ANU
Kuiam 291

Notes on Contributors 303

DEBRA ADELAIDE
Introduction

When you become a mother, or a parent, you find yourself doing a lot of things you could never have imagined doing before.

Certainly after my first—and second—child, I never imagined that I would be writing about it, let alone getting others to do so. But as every mother knows, your child is the most important, most extraordinary, most mind-blowing thing that has ever happened to you.

Many, many people are parents. But hardly anyone writes about their children. One reason is that children occupy an uneasy place in our collective psyche. We're expected to like the idea of them generally, but not to go overboard with our ardour; is this, I wonder, still a hangover of the terrible Victorian dictum that children should be seen and not heard? And then another reason,

1

of course, is that it's just too hard. It's often too hard to do anything much with children around, especially little children. Right now as I type this my four-year-old daughter is talking nonstop while ransacking my study for coloured pens, squandering sheet after sheet of paper, and pressing endless drawings onto me; I know that they are tokens of her love and therefore beyond all price, but at the same time I wish she wouldn't push them across the keyboard in front of me.

This, I've come to understand, and embrace (though reluctantly), is the amazing fact of parenthood: the extremes of emotion which a child provokes in you. I cannot think of any other relationship or situation in which you are alternately pummelled and caressed, thrown from the heights of elation one minute, to the screaming darkest depths of frustration and rage the next. And yet you survive . . . and your children thrive. This crazy paradox is one reason for this book, where once again women have written in vastly different ways about the exceptionally volatile emotional climate where motherlove flourishes like a sturdy perennial.

This book, like its predecessor, is on the one hand like a dream come true. To be a mother and a writer, and to tie those two crucial strands of your life together in a book (or two) seems the ultimate indulgence.

On the other hand, with these books I almost feel as

if some essential service is being offered, within the cultural void that seems to exist where this topic is concerned. It's like the books provide an outlet, a forum, even a soapbox, for writers who have long yearned to say something crucial about themselves and their children, and for readers who have desperately needed to read this.

What an egotistical claim! But then, after *Motherlove* was published, came constant comments: *I just loved your book . . . I couldn't put it down . . . I was having a baby and it was the only book I read in preparation for the birth . . . It made me cry, then laugh, then cry again . . . How come a book like this hasn't been done before? . . . I bought copies for my friends who were having babies . . .*

And then the letters, some of them quite extraordinary, and very, very moving. Like this:

I've read many thousands of wonderful books in my life, but this is the first time I've felt inspired to actually write and say thank you. I read Motherlove in less than 24 hours—not an easy task with a 13-month-old baby on my knee, but I just couldn't put it down.

Or this:

I recently read the very touching collection Motherlove and was enthralled by all 301 pages . . . It is one of the few books I could say I thoroughly enjoyed from cover to cover.

Or, most humbling of all, this from a woman who'd been dismayed to find herself unexpectedly pregnant:

When I came across your book, even as I read the introduction I cried. I cried because at last I was experiencing the feelings of longing, love, joy and peace for the baby in my womb . . . At last I had crossed over from feeling unhappy, disappointed, trapped and guilty because I felt no connection with my baby. I knew I wanted to feel maternal but reading your book was the trigger to experiencing these new emotions.

This last correspondent insisted that reading *Motherlove* had changed her life. The thought that a book you've done has changed people's lives is quite awesome, at once a burden as well as a delight. And yet the knowledge that the book reached out in this way only confirms all those instincts mentioned above: here were stories waiting to be told, and readers waiting to read them.

There were, too, other unexpected, delightful things. Like chance conversations: I'm phone-connected to the wrong person at a radio station, who says, *Oh you're the woman who did* Motherlove, *I just have to tell you how wonderful it is.* Or an encounter in a dark street outside a meeting: *Are you the* Motherlove *person? Thank you for that book!*

And then, the offers, from here, there and everywhere: *Look, I just have this story I've written, in case you're interested . . . If you're thinking of doing another book, I'd love to write something for it . . .* (Yes, we were thinking, but alas the new book was already pretty full . . .)

I report all this without a hint of blushing and in fact with a great deal of pride, because of course *Motherlove* and *Motherlove 2* are not just my books. They belong to the many contributors who have offered their passionate and moving, honest and eloquent, and funny and whimsical stories about what is clearly an endlessly fascinating and varied topic.

Motherlove—the word (contracted to one for a handy title) is like a long soft breath, reassuring in its assonance. Motherlove—the three unsibilated syllables move across the tongue and out the lips with remarkable ease. Is there anything more comforting, is there anything more secure, than a mother's love?

Of course, not all the mothering experience is as soft and cosy as that might suggest. Its starting point—conception—represents the ultimate moment of selfishness in the impulse to reproduce oneself; and its ending (wherever that may be) must expect nothing in return from children who never requested to be born. Mothering is also a difficult, tiring, frustrating, disappointing and ultimately quite thankless task. And the contributors to this book were certainly not expected to go all soft and gooey on the job. On the contrary, they were urged to be quite frank, not to hold back, and once again, to write about any aspect of the pregnancy/birth/baby/beyond process that interested them. But the one clear strong link across all these pieces is the sheer potency of a mother's love, in all its manifestations.

Motherlove 2 contains pieces about the change not just to lifestyle but to life and outlook that having a baby brings. There are pieces about the astonishing complexity and intensity of the emotions involved where babies and children are concerned. There are pieces that discuss or show the loneliness and mystery of the birthing experience. There is a story about the unforeseen difficulties in conceiving a baby. There are stories about relinquishing the mothering role, and surrendering much-loved children to the care of another. There is a piece that obliges us to accept a little-understood fact: that even when a baby dies, the mothering still goes on. There is a piece about something as simple, and yet as central, as a bed. There are diary stories, or ones that use journal entries, showing us the raw, unprocessed feelings at large both in the birthing room and in years afterwards.

There are pieces that talk about single motherhood (more than a few), about breastfeeding (quite a lot, actually), about relationships (some that fail, some that are strengthened), about sleep (or lack of it), about trying to get a child to read (and failing), and even pieces that talk about the unfashionable aspects of giving birth (epidurals, for instance, given the thumbs-up by more than one author). There's a bit of screaming. A bit of being utterly fed up. A bit of sheer, bloody exhaustion—and there's that too: blood. Not to mention a lot of milky confusion. And while we're onto the bodily fluids, there are, of course, the tears: joy, fatigue, rage, surrender . . . but mostly joy.

The more stories I read on this topic, the more I realise how endless the possibilities are and how—the experience being so undeniably life-centred, and life being what it is, an open-ended sort of thing—there'll always be another story that's different, another story worth reading. In one piece here, the author reminds us that hers is not fiction. *Reader*, she writes, *this is no story. Reader, this is my life.*

Readers, I think you might find in this book that this is *your* life too.

JANE CADZOW
Love that Moves the Sun

Five days after my father's birth, his mother propped herself up in her hospital bed and wrote a long, chatty letter to her husband. My grandfather worked for the trading company Burns Philp at remote Thursday Island, off the tip of north Queensland. Daisy, my grandmother, was a bright and beautiful 29-year-old who already had two daughters, aged six and seven. When she travelled south to Brisbane for her confinement, the two little girls went with her.

Daisy's letter is exuberant, filled with pride and happiness. She says the doctor had come to see her that morning and assured her she was recovering quickly. 'He looked at Billy and said he was a fine baby,' she writes. 'He remarked on his extreme fairness—as do the matron and others.'

She describes a plump, contented infant: 'He just wakes long enough to have a big meal and then collapses for another three or four hours. He's a perfect darling . . . I am looking forward to a four or five-year-old Billy, with fat limbs that I can dress in dear little sheer linen shirts and thick linen pants and a long white linen sou'wester hat, with white lace-up shoes and no socks.'

The letter is dated 31 July 1931. Daisy died on 8 August of a pulmonary embolus, a blood clot in the lung. My grandfather received the news by telegram.

I have been aware of this sad story all my life but now that I am a mother myself, it means more to me. My grandmother died suddenly. Had she time to think about it, I'm sure the worst part of dying would have been the feeling that she was abandoning her children. My father, her darling newborn, would never know what it was like to have a mother snuggle him on her lap, smother him with kisses, whisper words of comfort and encouragement in his ear. She would not be there to tie his shoelaces or bathe his grazed knees. He would have no memory of her. And her daughters. Leaving them would have broken her heart. Who would take them by the hand, teach them about the world?

Motherlove is so powerful and strange. On one hand, there is something wildly egocentric about it. In photographs taken immediately after the birth of my son, I beam as jubilantly as if I'd just won the New York Marathon. I brandish my baby like a trophy. *There! I did it!* Smug is the word that comes to mind, and I have noticed that other women with young children tend to exude a self-satisfied air: 'You may be a nuclear physicist/ winner of the Nobel Peace Prize/UN Secretary-General, but I am the mother of *this* miraculous creature. Eat your heart out.'

But a mother's love also has a selfless component. I know Daisy would have grieved more for her children than herself because I now know that's the way mothers are. Would I give my life to save my son's? Obviously. As would any mother (and most fathers) I know. I actually find it quite liberating that there's someone whose safety and welfare concern me so much more than my own. These days it's only when I am travelling with Gabriel that I fear plane and road crashes. When I'm by myself, I am quite devil-may-care. *We're going down? Have I time for one more gin and tonic?*

I worry more about him than I ever worried about myself. I have never been a particularly anxious person but when he was a baby, I tortured myself imagining accidents that could befall him. He was so small and vulnerable, the fragile centre of my universe. Even as he filled me with inexpressible joy, the terror that something could happen to him almost overwhelmed me.

My mother loves babies so much that she practically steals them from people in the street. She dotes on them and the feeling is mutual. Babies stop crying when she picks them up. They look trustingly into her eyes. She smiles back.

I have never been like that. Before I had one of my own, I had so little to do with people too young to walk and talk that I had never even taken a close look at one. They were all, well, *babies*. Small. Bald. No conversation. When friends gave birth I took flowers to the hospital then gratefully went home to my two-adult household and my very grown-up life as a journalist.

I loved my work as a feature writer. Loved my free time, too. Restaurants, movies, dinner parties, shopping, tennis, swimming, whole Saturdays spent reading the newspapers. It wasn't that I had decided against having a child. It was just that I was having such a good time that I kept postponing taking the step that I knew would turn my world upside down. Then in my mid-30s I started to identify with the woman in the cartoon who slaps her forehead and says, 'Oh no! I forgot to have a baby'. I decided that if I was going to do it, I had better get on with it.

Family and friends were taken aback when I told them I was pregnant. If they hadn't seen me as the maternal type, I wasn't convinced either. I was not the sort of mother-to-be who rushes around in a hormonal haze buying Laura Ashley curtains for the nursery. The very

words 'mother-to-be' made my toes curl with embarrassment. I didn't go to the antenatal classes: couldn't think
of anything worse than lolling about on beanbags with a
lot of other pregnant women, puffing and panting or
whatever the hell they did. I dutifully bought the
'Pregnancy, Birth and Baby' how-to manuals but guiltily
kept putting off reading them: there was always a newspaper
story or magazine article or novel of more immediate
interest.

When finally I skulked sheepishly into a department
store babywear section, I was appalled to find myself
surrounded by pastels and frills—jumpsuits adorned with
mint-green bunnies and bibs with 'Daddy's Girl' on the
front. Marvelling at the tackiness of it all, I bought a
bundle of no-nonsense white nappies, a few no-nonsense
white singlets and high-tailed it out of there. At home,
before I shoved the packages into a cupboard in the spare
room, I held up one of the singlets and caught my breath.
There is something amazing about a size 000 singlet. How
extraordinary that I would soon have a baby to put in it.

Still, I refused to be distracted from my work. I was
scheduled to start maternity leave the day the baby was
due. The day before, I finished writing my last story—a
profile of ABC presenter Kerry O'Brien, who had sportingly
kept a straight face when I lumbered hugely into his office
to interview him a couple of weeks earlier. I cleaned out
my desk, made some phone calls, felt a few twinges. That
evening, as the contractions came closer together, I

wondered briefly if I should have gone to the antenatal classes. Or at least read the books.

But in the end, giving birth came naturally. I was lucky. Next door a woman spent most of the night screaming at the top of her lungs, as if an axe-murderer were after her (I was curious, did *she* go to the classes?), but mine was a smooth, trouble-free delivery. David rubbed my back and gave me ice to suck. In the slow bits, he read *Scientific American*. Gabriel was born just before 11 the next morning.

Love. Instant, all-consuming love. Our beautiful baby. A perfect stranger yet utterly familiar. Gabriel.

The most wonderful day. Flowers. Champagne. Lots of phone calls—one of them from David to my office, where they were duly impressed by my promptness and efficiency: another deadline met. Outside my room, glorious spring sunshine. Inside, Cecilia Bartoli singing Mozart and Haydn; David had brought in the tape player. Gabriel lay beside my bed in his clear plastic hospital crib, a cotton blanket tucked around him, and slept peacefully. I looked closely at this baby. Examined the fluffy fair hair, the gentle tilt of his nose, his tiny pink ears, his minuscule fingernails.

A card arrived from a dear friend. Inside she had written a quotation from Dante Alighieri's *Divina Commedia*: *L'amor che move il sole e l'altre stelle*. 'Love that moves the sun and the other stars.' Yes.

In my grandmother's day, babies were corralled in big nurseries. Only at strictly timed intervals were they presented to their mothers. 'All the babies are awake and crying,' Daisy wrote. 'They wake, feed and sleep at almost exactly the same time. There are hours of dead quiet and then they begin with one breath. They are beautifully trained . . . '

Gabriel was with me all the time, feeding whenever it took his fancy. But the first night, he cried and cried. I paced backwards and forwards with him for what seemed like hours, wishing my mother were there to work her magic. He was disconsolate and I was so tired I was afraid I would drop him. Eventually I buzzed for a nurse, who wheeled him away so I could have a few hours' rest. I went to sleep wondering whether I would recognise him among the other babies when I collected him from the nursery the next morning.

Of course I did. I realised as I walked unerringly towards his crib that even in his hospital-issue swaddling, I would have known him from a hundred paces. I remembered that when I went to Japan I berated myself for ever having thought that the Japanese looked alike. How absurd. Now I wondered how I could have thought that babies looked the same.

Time passed. My mother came to stay. She had only to pick up Gabriel, her first grandchild, and he would stop crying. He looked trustingly into her eyes. She smiled back.

She went back to Brisbane, my maternity leave ended and, though I worked at home, life got horribly hectic. David's mother came to help us out; she and Gabriel were crazy about each other but I was racked with guilt and confusion. I loved my baby; I liked and needed my job. Could I do justice to both? In that first year, I sometimes doubted it. People I wanted to interview always seemed to call back when I was changing a nappy. Running to answer the phone one afternoon, I skidded on a tiled floor, hit my hand on the wall and broke a finger. There were several times when it all seemed much too hard, others when I was convinced my second name was Superwoman. Gradually we settled into a kind of routine.

Through it all, Gabriel retained his good humour. He is nearly three now, a gorgeous boy with firm opinions and an infectious laugh. When he was a baby, I wondered how people could be so cruel as to raise their voices at young children. Now I know. A two-year-old in a contrary mood will drive almost anyone to drink. *Another gin and tonic please*. David is endlessly patient; I'm not. Gabriel and I have some heated disagreements about things like teeth-cleaning (good) and toy-throwing (not good) but I can't stay cross for more than a few minutes. I am too much under his spell.

In polite conversation, we all play down our passion for our children, but the truth is, I am entranced by my son. Spotting him in a crowd of kids makes my heart lurch. Does this feeling ever wear off?

16

When he is a teenager he will no doubt refuse to be seen in public with me, but for the moment, he, too, is uncritically adoring. When I arrive to collect him on child-care days and he runs across the playground to give me a hug, it's the sort of reunion they do in slow-motion in B-grade movies. At night, he goes to sleep with his arms clasped around my neck. We are madly in love.

If I could have chosen, I would have had a daughter. I am one of four sisters; little boys (and big boys, for that matter) were a mystery to me. A girl seemed easier and more desirable in every way. When I discovered partway through my pregnancy that I was having a son, I was disappointed. Only mildly. Only for a couple of weeks. But how misguided I was. As soon as Gabriel was born, he was *exactly* what I wanted. And now I am so grateful to him for teaching me about the other half of the human race. (Some things about young males continue to puzzle me. What's the fascination with earth-moving equipment, for instance? Why are excavators, bulldozers and backhoes so thrilling?)

A few nights ago there was a report on the evening news about an attempt to reunite Rwandan families separated in the chaos of civil war. A photographer has had the brilliant idea of taking pictures of as many as possible of the thousands of children living in refugee camps. Their close-up portraits are displayed on walls in camps and population centres in the hope that some of their parents are alive and will come forward to claim them. As the television cameras rolled, a woman scanned the rows of small black faces. Then she shouted and staggered forward, overcome by emotion. She had seen her child.

Some of the children in the Rwandan photos looked sad. Some were smiling anxiously. The journalist doing the voice-over explained that the photographer had told them there was a chance that their mothers would see their pictures. This was why some clutched flowers. For their mothers.

I have a photograph of my father, taken when he was about my son's age. Pudgy limbs. Grave face. He seems to be wearing a linen shirt and shorts. On his head is a white sun hat—not a sou'wester, but close. As I look at the picture, my eyes fill with tears. If only Daisy could have seen him.

Sometimes, on warm evenings, Gabriel and I go into the garden and look up at the dark, glittering sky. Last night he told me that when he was big, he would get in a rocket and fly to the moon.

Love that moves the sun and the other stars. Yes, that's it.

SUE INGLETON
A Letter to Roxane

Alone, midnight, Perth Airport.

A small child in red bunny slippers cries her exhausted cry. The waah waah is aimed, torpedo-like, at her parents who sit spreadeagled above her, sipping Coke. Daahda, Mummee, the wail pierces my mind as her waah waah hiccoughs between their knees. She's tiny. I'd say she's not yet celebrated even one birthday. Across to my left sits an eight-year-old with her mother, who looks tired, but the child's alert, alert and bored. The television pumps out World of Sport, Formula One roars through the café area while 95 per cent of us avert our gaze and sigh for peace and quiet. I look behind and there's another. This one must be 12. Cool and aloof, her hair like pale cornsilk, beautifully braided, she sits with legs together, jeans ironed. My eight-year-old sprawls across the chrome chair, with her back to her mother, her straight brown hair tucked behind her ears, vagrantly sliding around her neck. She sprawls with considerable grace and beauty. My baby is in her mother's arms now, sucking on her bottle whilst Miss Ice Maiden, her hands caressing her pressed denim, stares pensively into the darkness where ghostly 747s stand like great white slugs, awaiting the electric charge.

I'm going home to my empty flat.

I have a room to rent in my two-bed flat. It's really half a house with a lovely old garden. 'Roxi, I've found the most brilliant house! Quick, come on, I'll drive you round and show you, quick! You can have a squizzy from the outside, we can move in in two weeks!'

'I can't *hurry*, Mum, I can't walk! Remember? My toe!!' Ah yes, she's crippled, ingrown toenail op, the third time for the same toe, goddam those doctors, never know what they're doing. The Intone Grownail her big brother used to call it. We sit outside number 94 in the car and stare at the house, taking possession. The mad, overgrown front garden boasts two limey-yellow wattles and three huge magnolia trees, white, pink and blood purple. 'It's huge! I got inside this afternoon, there's a garden at the back too, Gil can go mad.' We move in. Her room has the bay window and the view of the garden and the noise of the traffic, but being 12, she can sleep through anything. It's sunny and light, we strip the rotten wallpaper and she paints the walls—with a little help from her big sister—

20

then she covers them with pictures, shrines to Brad Pitt, Keanu Reeves, silverchair, Mettallica, Megadeath; my shrines were to Ricky Nelson, Elvis Presley, Troy Donahue, Crash Craddock and the Everly Brothers—we are very alike, my love child and I. That was three years ago.

My baby is staggering around with renewed energy, the parents are on the move, their plane to Sydney has been called. She's running ahead just barely holding the tip of her mother's hand, just barely touching the earth. You were walking at nine months, Roxi. You were walking and out of nappies; well, on the farm, nappies were a little superfluous. I was addicted to disposable dri-tots, which I chucked on the compost and covered in dirt. But it was easier and warm enough just to let you run around with nothing on. The terrible part was that, if you pooed on the ground, the dogs would eat it, nature's way of recycling, I insisted.

One more little cry of Dadda-dah and she's gone. Oh my heart, what would I give to have you back with me for one day, aged nine months! My true memories are confused with photos. Blue, blue eyes from my father, olive skin from your dad, blonde hair from the Nambucca sun. The joy and horror of the years in the caravan. Enid Blyton, you have no idea of the reality of Five Go Off In a Caravan. Roxi, you slept on the shelf beside our bed, the other two had bunks, and for the next five years, as they grew, they began to develop a stoop. Maudie's little corner had a picture on the wall beside her head, her

21

shrine was to Laura Ashley and the photo was of a bay window in a white bedroom with a window seat and flowery print cushions and curtains. It was the last thing she saw each night. By the time she turned 13 she had her own room and your dear dad had built her a window seat just like the one of her dreams. Five years in the 'van. I came to love the simple life—in the end, all I really wanted was a room with a door. The house grew up beside the 'van, the kids grew up inside the 'van till finally, one January, we all exploded. You and me and Dad moved into the shell of a home leaving the 'van to the big kids.

My eight-year-old has just strolled past, she's quite tiny, she moves to the window, she turns and stares at me. Sweet face, sweet age. You had a tough year when you were eight. That was the year that your dad and I split up. How easily we crash down the walls of love and trust, how blind we are to where they fall. How careless we become of responsibility. He cried in the kitchen, as he was trying to explain to you that he would be going to live in Sydney for a while. He cries easily, your dad, but this time it was a little different, for his heart was truly breaking, although at the time I had hardened to all that. I was relieved, I was strong, you would be too. Oh yes, you were strong, you ran out of the room and in shock we looked at each other, your dad and I, in dismay and shock, and then, just as suddenly, you were back, with a box of Kleenex which you handed to him, saying, 'Don't worry Dad'. But that little eight-year-old took on a mantle of pain and got fatter and fatter, covering up, needing something to put between you and a world of betrayal.

I can smell something sweet. It's the princess in the ironed jeans, she's walked past my chair with a glass of hot chocolate in her hands. She sits herself carefully and stirs the dark into the light. Her shoulders are thin and her small breasts are beginning to bud. You, my love, at 12, well now, you were full rounded and gorgeous. Girls get their periods so early these days. I was nearly 14 when I got mine. Maudie was 12 but you were only 11. 'Oh for heaven's sake, don't make a fuss,' you grimaced as I shrieked with delight. 'I don't want any *rituals*, Mum!' Maudie had had to suffer one of my rituals when she got hers. Candles and blessings which you had witnessed, and perhaps not quite understood. OK, OK. I'm just glad you decided to tell me. 'Well actually, I got it three days ago.' Whaat? And you didn't tell me? What did you do? 'I got some pads from Alex.' Oh great, your girlfriends know but I don't. 'Well I just didn't want you to make a fuss . . .'

Fiercely independent.

I'm in second stage labour. Sitting on the toilet, don't want to shit on the floor, my arms round Rick's neck, huge contractions. Kate's whispers are loud and gossipy in my brain, my sister's replies are jangling noise. 'Shut up,' I gasp. I breathe out, suck air in, close my eyes, Kate's camera hanging from her neck, she ushers herself and Sally out of the bathroom; breathe, breathe, eyes closed. I see myself, I am a small white bird flying flying my heart is bursting right behind me is the black tornado from the Wizard of Oz. Fly! Fly! My wings beat and beat my tail feathers are whipped by the edges of screaming spiralling blackness if I stop now I'll be sucked in doomed gone forever I fly I fly I beat my wings beat my wings. Got to get off now, get off. I stand up, 'Don't want the baby to drop in the dunny'. Rick half laughs, half serious. He gets me into the living room, plans for birthing in the bedroom have gone out the window. In the living room now, seated on the edge of the couch, my naked body huge with this baby—who is doing all the work, my midwife assures me—I have a soft cotton housecoat round my shoulders, I'm hot I'm hot, it's the middle of winter. The doctor hasn't arrived yet. I went into labour at 11 pm but my midwife, Lya—hugely pregnant herself—insists we don't need him yet. When he gets there, he's so tired, he goes to sleep on the floor and the birth progresses around him. Dylan and Maudie are woken up. 'Get them down now,' advises Lya, 'we don't want them to miss it.' Kate and John click away, she in colour, he in black and white, two experts with the Leica—two beloved friends, plus my sister, my midwife, my children and my lover and here's our love child coming through. Suddenly, just before dawn I become suspended in time. There is no more pain, no more breath, nothing. 'It's stopped,' I whisper to my audience. I stand up. My god I don't feel a thing! It's stopped. But there's a baby in there! I'm as still as the waters of Lake Placid. I put my hand between my legs and feel. Between my legs there is a round, hard surface. My child's head is right there. 'Oh my god, feel this, feel this!' I whisper to Rick. 'Oh my god, it's the head.' And then!—pounding from the Universe come the last, thrusting spasms of Birth. I'm on my knees, my arms around his neck, oh push pushh puusshhh! Arghh! There is no more pain, just surging energy, the force of Life bursting through me and then whoosh! 'Oh, it's a girl!' cries my sister. Of course it's a girl, says Myself, I've known all along it's a girl. I turn around and she's handed to me. I hold her wet and warm, blood and vernix, eyes open and staring into mine. Those eyes! They are black, black as night, black as the space between the stars. I am transfixed by those eyes, I see the universe, I'm in the deep space, there is no sound, but inside my head I hear her voice: 'This is what I am, this is where I come from and now I'm going back into this baby.' And the eyes, those great black pools, suddenly they zipped away, closed down, became pinpoints, became pupils, became the eyes of my daughter and she opened her mouth and called out, the umbilical cord still inside me, she called out, then Rick cut the cord, took her to him, his beloved daughter, his only child, his precious part of himself that I have given him. The sun had risen.

My plane is called. The mothers gather their daughters. I gather my laptop and handbag. We will be flying into the dawn. I will not sleep tonight. The moon is just past full. On the last full moon, it was a blue moon, oh once in a blue moon, that's when there are two full moons in one month, yes it was a blue moon as I sat in my car en route to a performance in Geelong, seven am, raining and cold, the night sky fading to lavender blue, the full moon still high in the sky, I sat and stared through the windscreen at the car in front. Its trailer, packed high with belongings, covered with a tarp and on the top, your bike, and in the car, you and your dad and his wife. I followed you as long as I could, then I turned off to the Westgate Bridge and you went north to live with your dad, to be safe, to be nurtured in a real family again, to finish your last two years of school, back up in the north where you began. My darling. I have crossed the abyss to do this. I have walked through the fire. I have torn open my heart but I know that I have done the right thing. I have, for the first time in my life, honoured myself, saved myself, and in doing this I have saved you and our love.

The full moon hovered in front of me as I ate up the Geelong road. The sun was coming up behind me when suddenly, flying out of the south came a great white bird. She swerved round and rode the air above me, then she veered towards the rising sun. A pelican. A lone pelican.

Mythical bird. They say that the female pelican will pierce her own breast to feed her young.

I am at peace now. This is for you, Roxane, with my love.

Debra Oswald
Caesarians, Storkmarks and Other People's Kids

I 'll begin dangerously—with what many people would consider heretical beliefs about childbirth. I suspect drug-free vaginal delivery is overrated. I reject the notion that my babies' method of entry into the world defines my feelings for them. I think the primacy of the mother's birth experience is disproportionate. I fear the natural birth movement has an excessive edge which imposes a new tyranny on women.

OK, this view might have something to do with the fact that both my sons were born by caesarian. Both were also conceived with the aid of fertility drugs, so their very existence has always felt like a surprising gift. I suppose we all view these matters through a lens manufactured by our personal circumstances.

The arrival of a baby is so intense and unsayable an

experience that, in an effort to handle those potent feelings, we leak them into the furniture and the details surrounding the birth. I'm sure the moment a baby slithers out between your legs onto your own lounge room floor, dimly lit and fragrant with incense, is a mind-blowing sensation. But so was the moment my son was lifted out of my belly and placed on my chest in an operating theatre. The feelings about that baby are mind-blowing and sacred rather than the room or the props or the process. But so much writing about natural birth seems to sanctify such details in a proscriptive and excluding way.

When my waters broke on our couch during a rerun of *I, Claudius*, it never occurred to me that I would end up meeting my baby in an operating theatre. I was attending the kind of birth classes where every couple was committed to home birth or birth centre, where words like 'epidural' were spoken in grim tones through thin, disapproving lips. I saw myself as robust, determinedly swinging my child-bearing hips.

It turned out I'm one of those women who would probably have perished a hundred years ago. Having my belly sliced open, numb and paralysed from the diaphragm down, was not the image I had always conjured of the birth. My guts being picked up and moved sideways was not the unique sensation I'd been hoping for. But the joy of holding a healthy baby blew all the potential disappointment out the operating theatre swing doors.

With both caesarians, the important moments were the same as those I'd read about in textbook descriptions of ecstatic natural births. The shiver of recognition when I saw their rumpled faces—'So, Joe, it was you in there all that time'. That strangely satisfying sense of myself as an animal, knowing that I had grown these creatures inside me. Staring endlessly at their sleeping faces, my ribcage gripped by that fierce surge of love. The milk-tingling feeling that swept through my breasts when they yelped.

I've got nothing to compare this with of course. And I'm sure natural birth is preferable. I do feel a pang of regret that I'll never know what that's like. But I've always been too suffused with joy in my two boys ever to indulge in regret.

Don't get me wrong. I'm not making apologies for the old interventionist system that views pregnancy as an illness, medicalises birth excessively, and disempowers women. And I don't mean to make light of the experiences of the many women who have terrible stories to tell and who can point out profound differences between their birth experiences.

Of course bad practices need to be challenged vigilantly, but in the lobbying process, a particular emphasis and mythologising language has developed which has a sharp edge. There are now hierarchies of birth experiences, a censorious tone, and a set of expectations on individuals which make many feel guilty and intimidated. This is surely an unintended by-product of a movement that set out to enable mothers to feel joyful and positive about themselves.

I refuse to feel like a birthing failure in the way I know many women do. I hear people speak almost furtively about their caesarians or other 'unnatural' births, treading carefully around a new orthodoxy that marks them as failures or the victims of medical con-jobs. I hear people speak about such things with shame and grief and I see writing about birth that fosters those responses. That's obscene. The arrival of a baby should never have shame or grief hovering around it.

The natural birth movement that began to empower women and push us free of male medical tyranny threatens to clamp down a new tyranny of its own. Let's fight for birth centres and home birth with safe backup, let's insist that women have full information and power over the process. But please, let's not bludgeon each other with fresh dogma and punitive expectations and shift the focus off those babies. A drug-free vaginal delivery is not the only access to the great primitive currents of childlove.

Both my babies were born with 'storkmarks'—a small red blotch at the base of the skull and a beak-shaped mark on their foreheads. Once I knew that these marks weren't permanent and would gradually fade, I became infatuated with them. Two fresh humans with their labels still on them.

Those first few days after a birth are immersed in such a weird haze of euphoria and panic mixed together. I remember the moment I saw Daniel spew up a small mouthful of bright blood. I lurched up and squawked into the corridor—'Someone help me, my baby's coughing up blood!' One of the sturdiest sisters marched in and said, 'Not to worry. That's your blood, dear'. And there was a rush of great relief, 'Oh, that's OK then'. I had sometimes hallucinated that the baby was sucking the life-blood out of me through my poor ravaged nipples, and it seemed he was.

It's strange that something as basic to survival as breastfeeding should be so susceptible to problems. It's not some instinctive skill—you need advice. And so many of us copped conflicting advice from each shift of nursing staff, each new wave frowning with disbelief at the methods recommended by the previous shift. I certainly remember the frustrated rage I felt when some pert-lipped 19-year-old delivered a singsong lecture about breastfeeding, while hot currents of pain were shooting through my nipples.

I also remember hanging out for the shift of the fantastic ginger-freckled New Zealand sister. She swung into my room on Day Four or so, when tiredness and whirling hormones had pulverised my confidence. 'How are you today?' she grinned. I immediately crumpled into tears, in the sub-cerebral way that one kind word can make you do. I don't think I managed to blubber out any sort of explanation. She clasped my hand. 'You're a good mother,' she said. 'Know that you're a good mother.'

It was like an injection of some instantaneously reviving drug. She had cut straight to the subtext—almost comic in its baldness and excess. She said exactly what I needed to hear. Even now I feel the rush of grateful tears when I think about her. It was an astonishingly intimate exchange between virtual strangers—the kind of sudden intimacy that you encounter so much when children are in the scene.

In those first few days, I was gripped by a passion to protect this helpless creature in my lap, and my brain fostered all kinds of odd paranoias. Each day I spent in hospital, my partner Richard visited us after work. But he would always come in so exhausted—shattered, it seemed—and fall asleep on the end of my bed. To begin with, I gave him heaps, naturally: how dare he plead tiredness when I was the new mother, awake half the night? Then I noticed brown splotches appearing on his forearms. He could never offer an explanation for the splotches—just mumble drowsily and nod off again. Why was he so sleepy, with mysterious brown skin lesions?

I begged him to see a doctor. During those howling lunatic hours in the middle of the night, I was convinced Richard must have some gruesome terminal disease and that the cruel hand of fate would render my newborn fatherless.

Coming home from hospital, I was shocked to see artefacts from my ancient former life—only a few days ago. Pre-baby existence now seemed alien and distant like some past life as a Pharoah's daughter. I had planned to spend the last weeks of the pregnancy cleaning out the old kitchen of the house and converting it into my office. Early labour meant the work was never started. And now my professional writing self was obliterated, drowned in breastmilk.

Then I noticed that the door of the would-be office had a huge red ribbon on it. Richard was smiling slyly. I pushed open the door to see my new office, created out of the shell of the demolished kitchen. Painted, furnished, curtained, with my old desk stripped and resurfaced. Perfect.

Already soggy with emotions and hormones, I burst into tears. Happy tears, I mean. My career as a writer was still alive—contained in that room—even if it might have to wait a while for me to use it. It was the best present Richard could ever have given me.

The mystery disease was now explained. He'd been getting up at dawn to work on the renovation before I came home from hospital, hence the exhaustion. And he'd used a dark stain on the desk, hence the brown splotches on his arms.

That summer after my first boy was born was probably the most uncomplicatedly happy time of my life. I'd met another new mother, Michele, at antenatal classes. She'd dripped litres of colostrum onto my kitchen benches in her four crazed weeks of pre-labour, so there was already a bond. Over that luxurious dreamy summer, we rolled around on rugs in the backyard sun with our kids. Drinking endless cups of tea, cooing at the babies, while the events and anxieties of the outside world were like some muffled noise offstage.

These days, there's never enough time. I'm a harried and neurotic writer, Michele's steaming through her last year of a medical degree, we've both had second children.

But there's a photo of us taken that summer, on my back verandah—a pair of blissed-out milky frumps, rejoicing in our elastic-waisted daks, cradling our babies like treasures with a pulse.

When Daniel was aged between one and two, we lived overseas, based in a company house in a middle-class dormitory suburb of London, but travelling around Britain and Europe a fair bit.

Travelling with a baby has obvious limitations. But it also throws open routes that libidinous 20-year-old back-packers and other childless travellers never follow. People strike up conversations with you when you have a toddler in tow. Even in the most tourist-battered town, where the locals regard visitors as irritating and of interest only for their wallets, children broker connections. Fractured conversations filtered through dictionaries, but lit up with beaming smiles.

In Germany, people would stop in the street to offer

Dan a sweet from the tin carried for the purpose of indulging kids. A Heidelberg bank manager hurled himself across the teller's counter to fuss over the baby and ply him with trinkets. We were shown around the district and invited home for a meal by a family with a toddler with whom we still exchange letters.

There was so often an automatic kinship with strangers when Dan was there. They recognised us—we were parents too. We knew this emotional landscape that they inhabited too. However vast the language and cultural differences might be, we had something profoundly in common.

Unfortunately, London was not the best place to be based with a small child. In the streets of London, children are ignored and often regarded as nuisances. It's OK to fuss over the dog of a passing stranger, but kids seem like some faintly embarrassing thing, rarely smiled at or spoken to.

In almost every other place on earth, children are seen as a treasure to be shared by everyone. There's something deeply sad and joyless about a culture that misses out on fully enjoying children, including other people's children, and even the children of tourists passing through. I hope we remember that in Australia.

I always feel more plugged into the human race when I take time to fuss over other people's kids. That slightly deranged woman behind you in the supermarket checkout queue pulling faces at your toddler is probably me. At the risk of sounding like one of those tiny books of feel-good aphorisms, grinning at a passing baby is an inexpensive way to give yourself a flush of delight.

I love holding friends' small babies, falling unconsciously into that rocking and patting rhythm again, feeling a rush of memory as they snuffle into my neck. And when circumstance and their parents' generosity make it possible, growing a special relationship with a child other than your own is like a bonus, a gift.

If having kids plugs us into humanity, it also often renders us hostage to fortune. When they're little, the protectiveness is simpler—an animal urge to shelter these vulnerable things from physical danger and to soothe immediate distress. As they get older, the complexity of the world they inhabit makes it harder.

Picking Daniel up from school one day, I realised he was in tears within seconds of shutting the car door. Some nasty manoeuvres in the jungle of Year 3 social politics. Thank Christ Dan was not the direct victim in this case. But he was still distressed—wanting to know why he couldn't be friends with the combination of kids he liked, why he was ridiculed for playing with the boy picked out to be the victim by the class bully.

I attempted some parental wisdom which was promptly rejected. 'And *don't* tell me stories about when you and Dad were little,' Dan sobbed. Fair enough. When you're in Year 3, stories of playground dramas from the Olden Days don't help much.

In the rear vision mirror, I glanced at his face, red and

puffy from crying. The storkmark had come up on his forehead, as it does when he's distressed or hot. That storkmark. Olympics projects, rock collections, knock-knock jokes and all his other eight-year-old sophistications vanished for a moment, and Daniel was my tiny newborn again.

And there was I sitting ineffectually behind the steering wheel, helpless to protect my baby from the nastiness and confusion in his world. What could I say ? People can be vicious sometimes. Watch carefully, protect yourself, try to behave honourably and generously, if in doubt be kind—but none of that is any guarantee that you won't cop it. I couldn't offer him much parental advice. Best I could do was remember, with piercing vividness, how bewildering school can be and offer my support for his struggles, offer my respect as one human being to another.

Cramming two children and two careers into one household can be hard going. Sometimes at our place, we barely stumble across the line at the end of the week before it starts again. The logistical and psychic split of the working parent is undeniable. But one of the many side benefits of having kids is the sanity-saving perspective they impose, whether we like it or not. A reminder that the distortions and urgencies and ego-structure of our working lives are not the only reality.

If I've had an excoriatingly terrible day at work, I still

have to come home and make dinner, run the bath, answer questions about sand dune formation, draw an acceptable pirate on the side of a cardboard box, gasp adequately over a merit certificate for Consistently Good Behaviour. At first it feels impossible. All I want to do is huddle under the doona in a vodka-soaked Festival of Self-Pity. But, like all working parents, I have to force myself to continue, go through the motions at least. And then there'll be a moment—a flurry of Dan's laughter or Joe's tongue stuck out in pirate-colouring concentration— that is so intensely real and immediate and important, that it sweeps away the Crisis of the Day. Or at least shoves it into a corner with a bit more perspective.

Most winter Saturdays I'm there with the other soccer parents. Thermoses in hand, we group on the sidelines, watching brightly coloured flocks of eight-year-old boys and girls. We soccer parents laugh at ourselves—getting so over-excited about a near-goal, wondering out loud if we should get lives of our own. We get to know other people's kids in the team—gasping about their courageous run or fumbled kick or frustrating but lovable tendency to vague off.

I scan the park and spot my small boy, Joe, at a meeting of the Little Brothers' Club—an unofficial alliance of four-year-old siblings. Roaming in a pack, they conclude that teetering over the edge of the wall into the waters of Iron Cove is not quite dangerous enough and head for the electrical substation.

Joe suddenly looks so grown up, striding across the grass, that it makes me wince. With the first child, we are so impatient, on the lookout for any hint of a developmental milestone, yearning for the first roll-over, first steps and first words, unknowingly wishing their babyhood away.

With the second or third child, we're not in such a hurry. All Joe's milestones passed with a faint groan of sadness from me. It felt more like the last crawl, the last breastfeed, the last babytalk, rather than the first anything. If I could bonsai him as he is right now, I'd consider it. But growing up is an urgent business for Joe. He assures me that he has to grow up so he can learn to drive. I have to respect that.

Meanwhile, the referee's last whistle goes and the soccer players swarm around the parents to gobble up orange quarters and praise. We parents are enveloped in that thick, salty fog of sweat particular to eight-year-olds en masse.

I don't know exactly how any of those kids was born— from their mother's womb untimely ripped, delivered into a warm bath in a rush of ecstasy, yanked out by forceps. Maybe if you asked their parents about the birth, they would have some regrets, things they are angry about or would prefer had gone differently. But huddled on the side of the soccer field with our gorgeous kids, the details of their births are thumpingly irrelevant to every one of those parents.

Dan is gasbagging to me, explaining some defence strategy he pulled off. He's still out of breath and red-hot from running. Hot enough that the storkmark shows through faintly on his forehead. He interrupts his blow-by-blow about the game and frowns at me, puzzled. He wants to know why I'm beaming at him in such a gormless way. That storkmark. My baby. That blazing love we feel for our kids that blows everything else away.

GRETEL KILLEEN
Mouse

My five-year-old daughter, Eppie, wants to get a home loan. She thinks it's a Federation house with a labrador and a pool.

We live on the cusp of inner-city Kings Cross, where the kids can't play outside in bare feet because of the litter of syringes. We have a rock band on one side, an Indian restaurant on the other, a half-way house across the road, and nearly everyone else in the street is gay. I can't knit, I can't cook, I'm not married and I'm not blonde. Don't tell anyone but we don't even have a Land Rover. We live a long, long way from Meadow Lea and Freedom Furniture.

* * *

I have this nightmare. I forget to put my clothes on. I'm running late, I get in my car and I drive as irresponsibly as I possibly can for no apparent reason while fiddling with the radio, slappin' on the lippy, flirting with the mobile, and doing a quick impression of Whitney Houston singing that all-time classic, *I Will Always Love You—oooo—oooh—oooh—ou*. Suddenly I'm pulled over by two women, one of whom looks remarkably like a cross between Bernard King and Tonia Todman, and the other like Prudence Winston, the head of the kindy P&C. In perfect harmony they ask me to show them my Mother's Licence.

I check the glovebox, where I find the gizzards of a Chokito bar and 17 unpaid parking fines. I check my handbag, where I find a broken yo-yo and a doll's head, and discover that I've lost my wallet. And I check under the car seats, where I discover my children. They're both dressed in their pyjamas, eating rubbish, picking their noses, drinking Coke and watching some violent television program which is somehow being transmitted via my rear vision mirror.

Bernard/Tonia and Prudence offer me a homemade muffin (which of course is not burnt), and they politely tell me to speak into a bag (one that Bernard/Tonia has crocheted herself). They ask me questions pertaining to stain removal, head lice, vasectomies, lamingtons and what to do with the mortifying discovery that your son can't read Japanese by the age of two even though he is obviously brilliant because he is tall for his age, ruggedly handsome and extremely clean behind the ears.

I say something wrong. They dress me in a brunch coat and send me to reform school, where I share a cell with my mother, and we whinge about men, eat singed chops and discuss Aunty Joan's foot problem for the rest of our lives while watching the *Midday* show, reading *Women's Weekly* and learning how to make the perfect sponge.

* * *

Basically there are three types of mothers: the *Naturals*, the *Know-Alls*, and the *Naives*. The *Naturals* are the girls who wanted dolls that wet their nappies, who sewed pantsuits for the cat and tied pink bows around favourite rocks in the garden and then invited the rocks to a tea party. Now that they're mothers the *Naturals* smile when they iron, wash whites whiter than white, and can make a Home and Garden award-winning meal out of a sock and a raw potato.

Know-Alls are the girls who put their names on their pencils and learned to tongue kiss from a book. They like dogs and chase them in public with a plastic bag and a washing up glove, but prefer cats because you can teach them to wee all day long in exactly the same spot. *Know-Alls* are still married and they say they're in love, but because they only have sex once a month they are forced to folk-art their houses.

Naives are the mothers who haven't got a clue and never ever will, just like me. Sometimes I wonder what my kids will say in therapy—'She made us wear skivvies, she couldn't boil an egg, the only time she ever sewed she stitched the power cord to the machine, our Barina smelt and so did our school lunches, and we never even had Osh Kosh.'

In an effort to learn about motherhood as rapidly as possible the first thing I did on discovering I was pregnant was book into a beginners' birth class. (Fortunately I knew the night I conceived because after months and months of trying I ended up dressing as my husband's golf bag one night, just to get his attention.)

And the second thing I did was tell my mother. I probably shouldn't have told her until after the birth, because sharing my pregnancy with my mum was akin to sitting naked in a pet shop window for nine months. But then again, if I'd waited, St Vincent de Paul would have missed out on two thousand, four hundred and fifty-one badly knitted booties.

So, who's more important?

To tell you the truth I didn't really appreciate Mum until I became a mum myself and I actually remember the moment the light of gratitude first shone. I was standing in the kitchen, pudgy, teary and exhausted, and I was consumed with an urge to ring her: 'Hi Mum, I just wanted to apologise if at any time over the past thirty years you thought I was rude and didn't appreciate you ... and to ask if you'd mind coming over and showing me how to burp the baby.'

Nowadays my mum helps me with the kids three afternoons a week. My kids call her 'banana head' and Mum being Mum, she answers. She still can't cook and she can't wash up, but she can kiss a sore bleeding pussy knee and magically make it better. And she can hug like a winter doona.

* * *

A single, childless thirty-something Greek friend of ours, Ulysses, wanted to know if his mother could hire my kids for a weekend—because she wanted some 'grandchildren' to play with. 'Play grandmother!' I said, with visions before my eyes of lollies, presents, late night magical stories and endless, boundless cuddles. 'I'm afraid that's going to cost her quite a lot, 'cause of the wear and tear on the kids.'

* * *

I wanted to say thank you to my mum for all her help, so I decided to take her away for a rest. But Dad's dependent on Mum and the kids are dependent on me, so we had to take all the things with us that Mum needed a rest from, i.e. the entire family. As predicted, no one got a rest because we spent the whole time hearing, 'I'm tired, I'm hungry, are we having fun yet?' ... and that was just from my father.

Sometimes I wonder about the nuclear family thing. I guess a husband can offer encouragement and support, but then again, so can Oprah. And my son gives me encouragement and support and, when she's not dressed up as a bride with no undies on, my daughter also tries to.

* * *

When Eppie was four she held my face in her tiny little hands, pulled me closer and whispered up my nose, 'I love you, dickhead'.

* * *

Between the two of them, my Eppie and Zeke have got the kid thing sussed. Recently I was completely exasperated and asked little Zeke how many times I'd have to tell him to clean his teeth and go to bed—and he answered 'five'.

* * *

I, on the other hand, do not understand a single zot about motherhood. All I know is that kids are like computers and if you've got a deadline, the system will break down. And I know that if you give kids chops they'll want sausages, that they'll wake every morning at 5.30 until you have a 7.30 meeting and then they'll sleep in till nine, that everyone else they have ever met has more fun, more toys, better clothes, a bigger TV and an entirely superior existence. Only last week Eppie announced that this is the worst life that she's ever had.

My son turns eight in a couple of months and I still get a shock when he calls me 'Mum'. I often think that I'm going to wake from a dream, I always feel like I'm playing grown-ups.

Sometimes I'm so tired I sit on the couch and cry. And my son and my daughter hold me close and kiss my tears and whisper the words that I say to them: 'Don't worry, it's OK, we love you, you're the greatest, you are the love of my life.' And then Eppie will sing a self-devised song called 'You are my favourite mummy', and do some ballet which for no reason at all ends in a somersault that careers her into the couch. And then she'll burst into tears, quickly recuperate and demand a 'cloud of a roar', which you'll understand is 'a round of applause'. And then Zeke will put on a yo-yo show just for Mummy and he'll do 'around the world' in the living room and the yo-yo will smash into the chandelier and break another bit off . . . and life will be all back to normal.

And then they'll fight about who's cleaned their teeth, who's done their hair, who's got their lunch, who's made their bed, who spilt their breakfast, who drew on Mummy's work, who's sitting in the front, who hit whom first, who said what and why they said it, who's got more mandarins in their lunch (which neither of them likes but which they compete over anyway) and which of the two of them Mummy loves most. 'Which of us do you love the most, Mummy?'—'I love you the most and I love you the most, too.'

I could never have imagined myself saying that.

This morning I woke up crying. I'd dreamt that a group of us were sheltering beneath an underground doorway: men, women and children. Suddenly a man entered and said that all children under eight were a hindrance to the group and had to be killed. Then he touched each of my children on the arm and I knew that they would die. And they knew they were going to die, and Eppie didn't seem to mind, but Zeke had fear in his dear, sweet, sensitive, trusting eyes and I held both my babies and we lay on the floor and I said to them, 'It's all right, wherever you go I will come to get you, I will always be with you, I will always find you, I will always love you. We are safe, I love you.'

* * *

At the moment we have a mouse under our house. It's too smart for the poison or a trap and we're trying to work out how to remove it. Eppie has suggested a plank from the sink that balances on a small ledge and leads to a bucket of water. On the plank will be a Tim Tam to entice the mouse to walk the plank, tip it and land in the bucket. (When she was four she took a dead beetle to school and told everyone it was our pet.) Zeke on the other hand did not see why the mouse should have a Tim Tam when he couldn't, and so he suggested a sign that read 'Happy Birthday Mouse ... free apple bobbing'.

As of this morning the mouse still hasn't been caught.

* * *

51

When Eppie was a baby she was woken in the night by two screaming possums fighting in the ceiling. We were alone, together in my bed, as always. She cried in my bed and I fed her. It was very dark. I had a torch, I changed her. I watched her. I was so tired. I was scared of the possums, I was scared of the dark, I was scared of the loneliness. I was scared she would wake her brother and the circus would begin. I was scared of her tears. I was scared of her fear. I was scared that whatever she needed I couldn't give her. I was scared that I wasn't a mother.

I watched her. I watched her pretty face and her hair trying to curl and her little arms raised as she fell back to sleep, and my fear stilled: I'd done it again, I'd calmed my baby and regained control and I felt like I'd got away with it one more time, but that next time I was bound to get caught.

I watched her, and she was quiet, and I went to lift her gently, not breathing for fear that I would wake her. And I put my arms under her little body. And I saw a funnel-web spider by her head.

I picked up the torch, raised it high and brought it down with a crash to crush the spider. And I killed it killed it killed it, and ground it into the white doona cover, a smear of brown and legs and blood, just a 'hair trying to curl' from my baby's head.

Last night, five years later, Eppie was wearing a floral bra and frilled floral skirt. I'd told her to dress in something warm for bed, and she'd dressed herself as Carmen

Miranda. Now, once again in my bed, because she's been sick, my daughter finally fell asleep. Her laboured breathing wheezed and strained, while her face of an angel perspired gently, after five years still the most beautiful sweet thing I have ever seen. I kissed her and she stretched her little legs and pushed me out of the bed. I tried to slide her back to her side, but every time I shifted she would occupy more space. At night kids grow extra arms and legs.

The doctor said it was asthma and I've just spent two entire nights rubbing her back, holding her tiny body and breathing with her, the way my mother used to do with me. But Eppie's better this morning and theoretically off to school, although at the moment the reality is that she's standing in the kitchen completely nude doing what appears to be a drawing of some simplistic underwater life form. She then announces that it's me.

'Thank you darling, that's beautiful.' (Positive reinforcement.) 'Now stop doing that and get ready for school.'

'Just a minute, Mummy, how do you spell Gretel?'

'Eppie can't you do this later?'

'Mum, please, how do you spell it?'

'G.r.e.t.e.l.'

'Say it slower.'

'Eppie, we're in a hurry.'

'Mu-u-m . . .'

(Now I'm thinking that it will take less time just to spell it out than to go through this charade, but then am

I giving in to her, and will she learn that all she has to do is whinge and cry and then she'll get what she wants and obviously grow up to be a serial killer ... or a hugely successful eastern suburbs wife?)

I repeat it to her slowly, but dress her as I spell (this way I fool myself that I'm winning the war).

And now it's five to nine and school's about to start and Zeke gives her my speech about selfishness blah blah blah and Eppie couldn't care two hoots. And finally she puts down her texta, takes her scrap of paper and marches proudly out of the house. Zeke and I grab the bags and follow her, ready to jump in the car. But Eppie's stopped again, just outside the door, and I'm telling her to quit dawdling, and she takes some sticky-tape from the back of her hand and proudly sticks her work on the wall for all the world to see:

'I love grtl eppie.'

And Zeke reads it and he's furious, and he takes a texta from deep in his bag and writes:

'I love her more, from Zeke.'

* * *

And when we get home late that afternoon there's been a further addition to the sign:

'And I love you all, love, the mouse.'

54

ROSIE SCOTT
Birth Diaries

These descriptions of my daughters' births were never intended for publication and are in fact extracts from my diary. I decided to publish them virtually untouched because although they are embarrassingly rough, they capture the sheer joyful intensity I felt at the time.

Twenty years later and somewhat more chastened about what motherhood means, I can smile at my idealism and naivety. It seems hard to imagine that I woke a baby on purpose, or tried to live up to the impossible burden of John Bowles's severe and inaccurate rules for mothering. Postnatal depression, sleepless nights and the teenage years were still in the future.

Nevertheless, these birth experiences remain among the most profound and formative of my life, and the memory of them is still as moving as when our daughters were born.

Josie
November 1974

The pain and 'bother' of pushing every time a contraction came—everyone exhorting me to push. Having to stick my legs in the air and bear down when all I wanted to do was sleep. Feeling the head bursting down as if it were in my bowels rather than my vagina—and then that strange unreal moment as the body of our daughter skidded out, slithery as a rubbery doll, limbs shining and tangled on the white table in front of me.

The amazement of it—seeing a whole live round baby suddenly 'be' there, where before there was nothing—the soft rounded greasy limbs, her little folded-in wrinkled bum pointing up at me as artlessly as a flower.

Danny's face—all I could see were his speaking eyes above the white mask, crying with joy, his voice breaking with the emotion of it. And then after they had made her cry and wrapped her up and given her to me I put her on the breast and she sucked there as if she had always known me. Tiny little face and dry skin, and Danny's loving voice and beautiful joyful eyes, and me just wanting to sleep with the pethidine whirling in my head and trying to fight gusts of weariness.

And the labour—at the beginning I felt as if I were in control—I counted and relaxed and it built up like an enormous wave, but I was afloat and not sinking into it even though I was being buffeted around. Then like an idiot I took some pethidine which made me go to sleep. When I woke, the contractions were slower and I felt unpleasantly drowsy as if my mind was far off trying to tell me something important but my body would not listen. Then being sick and feeling quite helpless against the pain, trying to listen to what Danny told me and the nurses kept telling me, only they were miles away and it was like trying to hear and understand through glass. The meaning only came through in dribs and drabs.

I can't really remember much except the weariness of having to bear down—everyone telling me to, when all I wanted to do was sleep. An English sister whom I took a dislike to kept telling me to breathe, while flashing her awful square false teeth. I remember the grinding pain and saying to Danny, 'This is a nightmare!' I found the hospital bed very uncomfortable and kept trying to squat on the floor.

And then there was Josie lying there with all the doctors, nurses and sisters clustered around making her breathe and me just seeing her tiny limbs and feeling in a dream. And my darling Danny always gentle and sweet. I woke from a sleep and he was just sitting there quietly— I remember telling him to go for a walk and he just smiled.

Josie—how different was she on the instant of passing through from her shadowy world to here? Did she still have that little Florentine mouth and stare around in that trusting solemn way, or did she silently cry? Or look at me with solemn suspicion, her mouth like a little rosebud, her beautiful, thoughtful little spirit shining through her eyes? I wonder what she thought about in there during the last few weeks—day after day in her little watery dark place. How I love her with such a powerful tenderness. (I once read a book written by John Bowles, and he said every baby was born only with love)—her love is so perfect I am afraid I could never love her enough in return. Her little rounded head curved above the blankets, her infinite trust, her crying always for something and me wanting only to be tender and gentle and understanding all the time. Not to get angry—holding her in the dark, hearing her little sucks and sighs at my breast, her hands clasped below her chin.

This morning I woke about three am in my new room, with just a lovely predawn light outside and the wooden houses opposite like stage sets. I kept trying to go back to sleep but wanted Josie to wake up. I could see her perfect little face—smooth forehead, fluff of black hair, those curly ornamental lips so fine as she slept, and the deep folds of her eyes and nose. And she kept making little snuffling sucking noises and moving her hands, even opening her eyes with a blue flash and closing them again tight shut. I woke her very gently and brought her into bed lying facing me. She lay there so unsurprised, trusting and solemn with her hands clasped peacefully, me watching her little head. I felt such a wave of tenderness for her— sometimes it is almost unbearable.

And then she had her suck, snuffling, and after she did her 'ar ya' noise which is a very peaceful form of Josie-crying. And then, all hunched against my breast, and with great stoicism, she began a whole series of hiccoughs which hicked on for a few minutes and shook her little frame. She sits huddled with her swaddling cloth partly over her head so she looks like a miniature and rather grotesque Arab peasant lady about to make some very gloomy pronouncement. When she is sleeping she looks as if she were smiling, like one of those Buddha statues where the whole face is smiling even if the lips are not. Another noise is a kind of little scream, like the one I imagine the pig doing in *Alice in Wonderland*. And when she hears noises she focuses on them with her long, considering blind stare.

If I have any sensuous recollection of Josie's first week of life, it will be of great masses of pink and white flowers, water glistening in a canister, oranges, grapes, cleanliness, a peaceful window with pale pink brocade curtains and the sun shining in on the cane chair for visitors. Josie's white bassinet with her little pink coverlet and her soft head. Masses of flowers—the softest, floppy, scented roses pink and white in a crystal vase, enormous fluffy white carnations, deep blonde roses, a dark pink delicate cyclamen, white and yellow daisies, and pure white papery sweet peas all fragile and delicate. This peaceful room with my baby daughter sleeping beside me and the hum of the hospital. Waking at night to her plaintive little cry and holding her warm wet body, smelling her most beautiful skin and little whorls of dark hair against my mouth, and her wrinkled hands, her nuzzling mouth. Peace in late afternoon sun through the window and my mother sitting on the cane chair, cleanliness, purity. Danny gazing at our child and my breasts brimming over.

Bella
January 1977

I woke to this incredible knock or thump to my pelvic floor, like someone tapping me hard with a stick. It was kind of imperative and blind and seemed to act like a catalyst because the pains started straight away. They were very intense and agonising but I felt in control and basically comfortable. I was naked on the double bed, and that in itself felt good—Danny beside me putting up with my nastiness. It all happened so fast that when Caroline arrived, she just had to touch my brow and it calmed me down. I will always remember the touch of her soft cool hands relaxing me. It was really nice having Jo too— luckily they all arrived quickly because pretty soon the pains came every minute.

The transition stage came and it was unbearable. Then lying on the bed, I started to feel the sensation I missed out on with Josie—the most extraordinary splitting sensation—my whole stomach was being stretched and pulled, it kept coming and receding as the baby passed slowly down my vagina. I felt as if I would never get her out without breaking in two. Jo and Danny were supporting me on either side telling me to push, and then the head crowned and Caroline told me to pant and I just did. I was so proud of that, that I didn't push her head out but just panted it through. They held up a mirror for me, I was so busy panting I didn't see, until suddenly this great sleeping head came out all covered in white vernix, sticking out between my legs. I leaned over and slid her out of my own body and had her beautiful little soft form lying there all warm and wet and pulsating between my breasts. The feel of her body was incredibly sensuous, a big sigh of relief. Danny in tears of joy and cutting the cord. Caroline showing us the placenta, Jo such a nice presence, and Bella herself with only one little cry breathing immediately, such was the ease and joy of her birth. She sucked with incredible force straightaway, her tiny face all swollen, her little soft blood and mucus-streaked body so perfect.

The dawn was just coming—a beautiful confusion with cups of tea, Dick's incredulous face, peering in at the small baby on my breast, her birth so gentle it had not even woken him. Everyone bustling about and me with my sweet Bella cuddled up on me feeling such relief and release. To me it was the most perfect birth—no stitches or drugs or lack of control. It just happened, the clichéd natural birth became real to me when I realised how natural it is if all is well. Four hours of labour, our baby born and breathing and sucking and immediately loved and cuddled. Little Bella arrived like a gift, and the grey early dawn and the birth of our child on the high bed will always be a happy memory.

Now at home here back on the island, moving through the day in a kind of haze, beautiful blue February days, my body already feels back to normal again. Cuddling my little wrinkled wise Bella all pink and passive and lolling with her tiny blue considering eyes peering around with an air of ancient resigned wisdom, her hands fluttering in ceaseless motion.

Bella with her two-days-old smile, a floppy toothless affair, infinitely endearing. Sitting in the sun with her, both of us dozing in the warmth, her soft little head all drooping, whorled with soft fine mousy hair. While I was feeding her I caught her looking at me with a really quizzical expression, a faint frown on her face. As if she were seeing me for the first time, as opposed to the breast she had just been sucking. She is wearing her little purple cardigan, her blue eyes bright. She smiles up eagerly at me, her whole self animated as if I were the world to her—my presence alone brings her to life. Cuddling her is a warm electric thing—she still feels part of me to the point where I cannot leave her crying. Just now hanging up the nappies I left her for a few minutes in her cot. Her crying was like an ache. I had to run back and when I bent over her and she saw me, the relief in that incredibly human knowing little face shone out in her beautiful gummy smile—I couldn't hug her beloved sturdy little body hard enough. She is so beautiful, with a little domed forehead, wide apart blue eyes and curly little lips. She is bigger than Josie was with soft little fat arms and an incredibly gentle demeanour. Sleeping in her cradle she looks like a tiny perfect doll. She has long thin tapering fingers which move like anemones, and a very serious expression. When she is lying in her yellow bath she is like a Buddha, all smiling, loving, calm, her body glistening in the water. She always trusts us.

Her time of birth primal, with the candlelight giving way to the dawn coming through the high windows. She arrived at dawn, her serene presence immediately felt because she didn't even cry, just made this little sound, her body sliding out, that incredible closeness as I held her to my naked skin, surrounded by my husband, sister and our wonderful midwife—later my father and Josie peeping into the room in surprise. But holding Bella so lovely, Danny and I in tears of joy in the high bed in familiar surroundings, without drugs or tense hospital feeling. Bella not made to cry, but snuggling into me as if she had always been there, her own father cutting the cord, and holding her too, minutes after her birth. Bella arriving on earth with such style, a kind of quiet mirth in her as if she immediately liked what she saw. Received into the world in the quiet old-fashioned upstairs room facing towards Maungawhau, the extinct volcano, in her grandfather's house.

Nestled in amongst us all a few hours after her arrival: father, mother, sister, aunt, grandmother and grandfather there to receive and love her, celebrate her birth. It felt like an age-old, primal ritual, far older than the one now played out in sterile white hospital rooms, exactly right for our beautiful Bella's arrival.

To My Daughters

Your heartbeats come strongly through my skin
At this mysterious time, when all around you
Blood and darkness, the terrible beating of my heart.
My secret, silent child drowned in the dark
Tiny astronaut weaving and plunging in my inner space.

Small, exhausted, elderly, you dream of unknown lands,
and wait your turn. You sigh and move—
Perhaps you know I love you already.

URSULA DUBOSARSKY
Alone Like a Stone

When my mother went into labour with her fourth child, my brothers and I were sent away on a train to stay with our wicked auntie Barbara.

This was years ago, when it was common practice to have a midwife in to live with the family for the weeks prior to and following the birth. My mother had a woman called Glenda, which was a strange name then and I don't think she was quite normal, even for a midwife. But a great deal too much importance is attached to being normal, isn't it? What did it matter that Glenda hardly ever swallowed her food, but spat it out after chewing, laying it neatly in masticated piles on the side of her plate? What did it matter that she sang herself to sleep every night in the 'spare room' (although it was never that) with marching songs in foreign languages, interrupted unnervingly from time to time by bursts of peculiar laughter, which we, all in our own beds, lay waiting for in the darkness? What did it matter . . . ? Oh, enough of Glenda's oddities.

Well, not quite enough. Poor Glenda was made irritating by God or nature. She must have been at least 50 but she wore her fair hair in plaits with little tartan ribbons, in remembrance of some distant or not-so-distant Scottish ancestor who was slaughtered while kneeling at prayer in a highland forest. Her most onerous prenatal duty was to take toast and a glass of milk in to my mother for breakfast in bed each morning. Even this, I suspect, was a kindness on my mother's part, to give Glenda something to do, rather than mope about dolefully waiting for the baby to come. An unoccupied midwife is a melancholy sight, especially for the failing mother-to-be. Glenda would stand at the open window, gazing out with yearning eyes, as if the baby would arrive any moment by horse and coach, muttering to herself, 'Where is de baby? Where is de baby?' Glenda always said 'de' when she used the word 'baby', as though she had been lectured in the science of midwifery by a Scandinavian, and had never managed to shake it off. In all other instances she pronounced 'the' without any trouble at all. It was, in any case, a particularly ridiculous thing to say, as one look at my huge mother made it clear that the baby could only be in one place.

Glenda had not, I believe, delivered that many babies. She was what you might these days call 'underemployed', living on a dreadful rusty and splintery farm with her dangerously elderly grandmother in constant, excited anticipation of my mother's next pregnancy, and it had been over 10 years since I was born. On reflection now, I wonder if she really was a midwife, or if, like many things that made their way into our family home, it was simply a matter of being cheap and available; or in Glenda's case, free and available. I think my mother probably felt that she could deliver a baby perfectly well by herself, and again it was out of a sense of kindness and obligation that she called upon Glenda's services. Most of my mother's actions were performed out of a sense of kindness and obligation, old-fashioned virtues even then— probably old-fashioned even in the days of the Roman poets, of whom she was particularly fond. Unlikely as it may sound, my mother could often be seen with a copy of the *Georgics* on her high protruding lap, giggling away to herself, although what she found humorous about the life cycle of the bee is hard to imagine.

How long the days were, as we waited for mother's baby! It was the school holidays, so we were all at home. My brothers and I were each of us only a year apart, but they did not waste their time talking to me, although they entertained each other very well—setting up great papier-mâché landscapes of Belgium and re-enacting the various battles of the Great War with dozens of little tin soldiers. They had, to be fair, asked me if I wanted to play—I could be one of the Angels of Mons.

'I don't want to be an optical illusion!' I complained, reasonably enough.

'It wasn't an optical illusion,' retorted Matthew, affronted. 'It was a religious vision.' Which was hardly more inviting. So I abandoned them and sauntered about the house, pathetically humming tunes I knew from *Allen's Community Song Book*. My mother lay in bed all day, Glenda swept the house, and my father sat at his tilted desk by the window drawing maps on greasy grey paper. This is what he did for a living. They were not, alas, dramatic maps of the jungles of Indonesia, but rather prosaic charts of inland river systems and fields of arable land. My father was an invalid, he had cancer of the lung, so he had to work at home.

Unlike my brothers, whose blond heads were full of war, I thought a great deal about the coming baby. I did not know much about the processes of birth, but I knew from reading *David Copperfield* that it took a long time. I asked Glenda how many hours my own birth had been, but she just looked sick and said, 'Please, don't talk about it!' which is certainly not what midwives are taught to say these days, and cannot have been terribly encouraging for my poor mother. But later, when it was dark, and my brothers lay asleep next to me in bed, she filled me in. Blood, tearing tissue, screams, umbilical cords a mile long, great throbbing placentas sitting on the sheets as though with a mind of their own . . . I was born with the cord around my neck, Glenda told me, and she screamed out unhelpfully to my mother—'De baby is dead! De baby is dead!'—thinking that I had suffocated, but my mother leaned forward and somehow untangled me and there I was, pink and weeping and alive.

'You had such big feet,' Glenda whispered, as if it was some kind of ill omen—and who knows, perhaps it was in Scotland? 'I said to your mother, just look at those feet!'

'And what did she say?' Did large feet mean you were destined to be drowned or hung or persecuted across seven continents?

'She fainted,' replied Glenda solemnly.

How I wanted the baby to come! Although at the same time I didn't at all, because I knew it meant immediate banishment to auntie Barbara's, far away on a train. If it was dull at home, it would be even duller there. Auntie Barbara only had two books in the whole house—*Diana of the Crossroads* and *Nick Manaloff's Spanish Guitar Method*, which you could hardly call a book. To play with, all she had was a pack of cards with the jokers missing.

But waiting was worse. I used to steal up to my mother's bed when Glenda was sweeping, which was almost all the time in our dusty house. My mother lay on her back on top of the bedclothes, so fat, with her book, smiling secretly to herself as she mouthed the Latin syllables. I lay down next to her, thinking, listening to the sound of the broom, up and down, up and down. A baby! There was a baby in the room, listening with me. There was a person inside my own mother, a small lonely person. Soon the person would be coming out. Would my mother die? My father was going to die, that was clear. He coughed and coughed, all day and all night and had done so, it seemed like, for months. I wished he would stop. Would my mother die too?

It was breakfast time when it finally happened. Nowadays children eat cornflakes and drink orange juice for breakfast, but then such foods were for nudists or health cranks. We ate toast and homemade lemon marmalade, full of peel and seeds. Glenda came rushing in with wild eyes, and seized my father's hand by the fingers, shaking them up and down, which looked rather painful.

'It's de baby!' she cried. 'De baby is coming!'

'Well, at last!' said my father, pale, trying to look pleased.

My brothers and I exchanged glances, like soldiers whose numbers have finally come around. We had to seize our guns, pull on our hats and run out amidst the cannon fire.

My father followed Glenda out, hunched. I think he may have preferred to be sent to wicked auntie Barbara's as well, but he had his role to fill, to wait in the living room, to keep Glenda's spirits up, as she might well become hysterical if things did not go as she wished.

We went to our room to gather our bits and pieces. I

packed my school satchel with the necessary clothes and a magnifying glass, some paper and envelopes and my school reader. Our father came to the bedroom door and looked at us miserably.

'I wish you weren't going!' he said, almost crying, because my father was a bit of a baby, and Matthew had to go over and slap his shoulder and tell him everything would be all right and it would all be over before he knew it. My father coughed and dried his eyes. 'Come and say goodbye to your mother,' he said, taking my hand. He was an invalid, but his grip was strong. His fingertips were stained in red ink from his map drawing, reminding me of an illustration of a Hindu bride I had seen in the school encyclopaedia.

I was naturally nervous about seeing my mother in a labouring condition. I had supposed that once labour began she would be beyond communication, and the bed would already be covered with blood and body parts. Could she speak? Would she recognise me? My father led me down the hall to their bedroom, Matthew and Mark having run on ahead—they were not apprehensive, of birth or death or anything else, it seemed. Sometimes my brothers seemed to me like sprites of some kind, not human, but vain and immortal. They both had fair hair, so fair it was almost white. They were kissing her when I got there—she was lying in bed on her side now, covered in blankets. Glenda was trying to lower or raise—it was hard to tell with Glenda—the curtains at the window above her head. I suppose it gave her something to do. Pain came and left my mother's face, and came again. My father took her hand. I leaned down and kissed her goodbye.

'Soon you'll have a little brother or sister,' she murmured, but I must say she looked as disbelieving as I felt. How could there be two lives where now there was one?

On the wall opposite the bed hung one of my father's framed maps, entitled: 'Northern Tablelands River System'. I hoped that my own husband, when the time came, might provide some more romantic decoration than that, but I suppose my father was proud of it, and it was very finely drawn in soothing greys and yellows. Perhaps my mother would gain strength from it as she cast her eyes about the room in an agony of labour.

Fortunately she did not say, 'Be good for auntie Barbara'—my mother never said that kind of thing. And it is more than likely by that stage she didn't especially care if we were good for auntie Barbara or not. Matthew and Mark were eager to leave, I wanted to stay. My father led me out of the room by the hand as firmly as he had led me in. We went down to the kitchen to cut cheese sandwiches for the train trip. The bread was stale and the cheese slightly old, but my father seemed keen not to send us out with nothing.

'Once when I was a boy,' he said, reminiscing as he cut the bread, 'I arrived at school without my lunch! Imagine!'

'Couldn't you ask someone else to give you something?' I suggested, practically. I had on several occasions forgotten to take my own lunch to school and had not gone hungry.

'I should have,' agreed my father, sheepish. 'But I was shy. I didn't want to tell anyone. And I was so hungry!'

My poor father was very easily given to tears, and I could see some were on their way. I quickly interrupted them. 'You must have enjoyed your dinner that night.'

But my father was frowning, as if trying to puzzle something out. 'Actually,' he said, in a confessional tone, 'on the way home, I ate some nasturtium leaves, growing in the front garden of a house we used to pass by. It was a huge plant, I didn't think anyone would mind.'

'What did they taste like?'

My father bobbed his head from side to side. 'Oh well, you know what it's like when you're hungry, you don't notice, really.'

I thought that I would have noticed nasturtium leaves.

My father lowered his voice. 'Then as I was eating them, I saw a very strange woman looking at me out the window of her house.'

'What was so strange about her?' How could someone communicate strangeness merely by looking out a window?

'She was completely naked,' said my father, mystified. 'It was a very strange thing, you know.'

Now I pictured my father, the hungry schoolboy, mouth full of nasturtiums, being stared at through a window by a naked woman. I did not know what to think.

'Did you know who she was?' I asked.

My father shook his head and shrugged. 'Life is full of mysteries!' he said blandly. 'Anyway, I never forgot my lunch again.'

I don't suppose you would, I thought. He wrapped up the unappetising cheese sandwiches in newspaper.

'We'd better be heading off,' he said, patting my shoulder.

My father walked us to the station. I was shocked— what if the baby was born while he was out? But this did not seem to cross his mind. The road from our house was not tarred, and our shoes became covered with brown dust, and my father looked down at them several times, saying, 'Oh dear', but we kept on walking just the same.

We were the only people on the platform and it was hot. Matthew and Mark threw pebbles down onto the tracks, aiming for the sleepers, and my father coughed and we waited for him to catch his breath. He bought us each a return ticket but I felt as if we were crossing the Styx into the afterlife.

'Well, boys, Matthew, Mark.' Our father shook hands with each son as we stood on the platform. 'Look after your sister,' he added mechanically, and kissed me.

My brothers did not answer—they seemed neither nervous nor impressed. I suppose they had been through it all before when I was born, although they could not possibly remember it, as we were each only a year apart.

Matthew was actually still on the breast at Mark's birth, but a triumphant auntie Barbara sent him back after the prescribed two weeks 'fully weaned'. She boasted of it often, in a rather chilling way.

When the train pulled out, I'm afraid we scarcely glanced back at our father, waving, lonely, slightly comical, doubtless dreading his return home to where the great apocalyptic event was now taking place.

'At last!' said Matthew, and he and Mark smiled at each other, in the beautiful way only young boys can smile. They had stuffed their pockets full of paper and soldiers and rubber bands which they started to flick about the carriage.

I wondered about my mother—was our baby out yet? I pictured Glenda raising the child to the sky in bloody and triumphant hands, the blue serpentine cord reaching on and on into those terrible internal depths. Glenda would cry out, 'De Baby! De Baby!' and then drop it on the ground, babies being such slippery things.

But then my mother would take charge and leap out of bed and masterfully catch it just before it was dashed to pieces, wrapping it up in a rush of swaddling so that only the eyes were visible, dark, round and shocked.

And those eyes would stare out at my mother, accusingly. How had this happened? After months of being together, beating blood and soft rolling bones, now they were apart, forever. The infant was alone. So suddenly alone. Alone, like a stone, in the New World.

A rubber band pinged me on the cheek. I bent down, picked it up from the floor of the carriage and swallowed it. Mark whooped with pleasure and pinged me again, but I would not eat any more rubber bands that day.

MARGARET SIMONS
Why Clare is Not a Yahoo

Five months ago I became the mother of Clare, the warm little girl who is lying on the rug by my side as I write this. She has my eyes, and her father's sticky-out ears. She smells of sweet, vital animal, of earth and milk. She has just learned to play with a rattle. Every now and then she drops it, and I have to lean down to pick it up.

I used to think I needed uninterrupted time to write. Now I find that the mind can be like a slideshow—a series of stills, with a jerky break between each one. In flashes, then, ideas come together in ways that they didn't before, and so I find myself thinking about motherhood, and then about Buridan's ass.

Buridan was a French scholastic philosopher who died in 1360. He is remembered because he was reputed (though wrongly) to be the inventor of a fable about an ass which, placed exactly between two haystacks that were in every respect equal, starved to death because there was no reason to choose.

It seems that motherhood is about being in between, and mothers and babies could so easily waste away trying to choose how to be, and what to do.

Mothers dwell between the primal and the civilised. My waters broke in a gourmet pizza restaurant. I had just finished eating a pizza with basil leaves and char-grilled Thai chicken. The restaurant was called, ironically, Terra Firma, and it had terracotta tiles on the floor. The intended image was of earthy, peasanty things, but I still felt obliged to rush for the toilet to hide what had happened.

Mothers dwell between the private and the public. Clare exists in the domestic. She is a person who has not yet unfurled into the world. Nobody understands her cries as well as we do, or knows or cares about her smell, or her smile, or the consistency of her shit, as much as we do. Nobody else is wrapped up in her wet little mouth, her little lungs full of tiny air sacs, her little chambered heart, her little stomach—all her organs working marvellously. Little hands. Fingers in my mouth. I chew her nails to keep them short. We do these things quietly, privately. It concerns no one but us.

Yet I walk into my local bookshop and there is a shelf of books of mother care advice. They contradict each other, and each is written in the most uncompromising terms. This is how we know that motherhood only seems private. People don't bother to write propaganda about private things. They write propaganda about politics.

* * *

The fable of Buridan's ass is a story of the ridiculous. It is a story about the uselessness of logic, when it leaves you unable to make a choice. It is also a macabre story. I imagine the ass starving, becoming gaunt, then a corpse, then bones, while the haystacks sit smugly on either side. Imagine how the ass must have felt. Imagine the anxiety of starving in the middle.

Motherhood is an underground activity. I work as a journalist. This means I can work from home and look after Clare as well, but when I ring important men I hide the fact that I have a baby on the floor of my study. Her morning nap normally lasts half an hour. I use the time to call a politician, and make interview appointments with two captains of industry. On the telephone, I sound as though I am wearing a suit and sitting in an office, instead of wearing a T-shirt splattered with milk, a bra still undone from the last feed and tracksuit pants slightly damp on the knee.

Clare's father, Warwick, takes her out so I can concentrate, but I miss her. I think of the way she swings her legs up when I change her nappy, waving her little pink fanny at the world as she reaches for her toes. I think about the way she cries, her mouth a grumpy ripple like a cartoon drawing, and her eyebrows standing out white against her red face. Gargoyle features, I call her when she cries. I can afford to joke since she is a happy baby, and these days I know I can comfort her.

In the very last stages of my labour, the obstetrician said, 'One more push like that, Margaret, and you'll have your baby.'

I could feel her coming down out of me like a watermelon. I could hear the pad pad of her heart on the monitor. My mother and Warwick were there, urging me on, gazing between my legs for the first sight of her, and the thought flashed across my mind, mucking up my next push, 'Hang on, do I want a baby?' Then with a slither she was out, and moments later was on my chest, and for the first time I saw that newborn face, so serious because it hadn't yet learned to smile, and I fell in love. I turned to Warwick and said, 'Ah. Making babies. Let's do it again.' Or at least, that is what they tell me I said. I don't remember saying it. All I remember is that everyone was laughing at me.

For three days I was a powerful woman. There was nothing I could not do. Intoxicated, I had my mother bring me a tape recorder because I wanted to get down all the things I was going to write about giving birth. I wanted to tell about the moment when, trying to writhe away from the back pain, I was swinging from the bar over the bed. I am a very big woman. I must have looked like a great human ape.

I wanted to write about how in the final stages, when I was pushing a new life into the world, I could hear the midwives talking about staffing shortages.

'Too many people. Too much talk,' I said.

'Oh well, I'll go away,' the obstetrician said.

'No. *You* know what you're doing,' I snapped and at once felt bad because I hadn't meant it that way. It was the midwives who had got me this far. They knew what they were doing too, but the next contraction was on me before I could apologise.

For three days I was euphoric, talking into my tape recorder, loving Clare, feeling the primal strength and the civilised urge to write it all down.

Then I got homesick.

Clare had jaundice. Since the third day of her life she had been yellow-skinned and now yellow had crept in around the corners of her eyes. I had been told not to worry. It was normal and would disappear, they said, though it might make her sleepy. Because of the jaundice, I should feed her at least every three hours. If necessary, I should wake her up to feed.

Feeding was not going well. In the middle of the night, Clare would suck, then come off the breast and scream. It took me three hours to feed her, and then I slept only to be woken because it was breakfast time. Giving birth had been a matter of letting go. My body knew what to do. Nobody had told me that breastfeeding was different, that it was something you had to learn.

On the morning I was discharged I was packed and ready to go, itching to be home, but we had to wait for the paediatrician to check Clare. Hours later, he came. He took a blood sample for her jaundice, and weighed her. She had lost weight. A midwife remarked in passing, 'We like to see them put on weight before we let them go'. More waiting. Warwick loaded my cases into the car. Then the results of the jaundice tests came back. 'It's higher than we expected,' the midwife said. 'He said you could stay in for a day and have them done again, but I said you were almost out the door . . . ' and we were.

Home with this tiny, serious girl who still had to learn how to smile. She slept for four to five hours at a time, if I let her, but as instructed I woke her by the clock, and she was tired and I was tired and we struggled together with my great weighty breasts. Latch on. Come off. Scream. Then she slept, but I couldn't. I lay and listened to her breathe.

Post-baby blues is a deceptive term. What I felt was not so much depression, as heightened anxiety. In the hollow hours of the morning those two pieces of information at the hospital came back to me. 'Losing weight. Jaundice worse than expected.' I looked at the clock. I woke her and we struggled again. Sitting there with her, so bound up with her and so alone, I remembered another piece of advice. The obstetrician had said: 'Never wake a sleeping baby.' Should I wake her, or should I let her sleep? It seemed like a life and death decision. Buridan's ass. Except I thought it was Clare who was starving.

It was now two nights since I had slept. I cuddled up to Warwick, so tense I could hardly breathe. Having this child was the worst thing I had ever done. I couldn't look after her. She would die in my care. How could I get out of this? I thought about leaving that warm bed, walking to the nearby train line . . .

'I'm having thoughts that frighten me,' I whispered to Warwick.

Clare was sleeping quietly, snuffling gently. I was so tense I couldn't lie still. He said, 'Oh Meg. What are you doing to yourself?' Then he gave in to his own exhaustion and slept, and I spent the night rigid, hanging onto him.

When she woke, we got out the breast pump I had bought for when I would go back to work. I watched my nipple being drawn into the whirring machine while the little warm animal girl curled in Warwick's arms. We fed her the milk by bottle, and I knew from all my reading that by doing this we were making the problem worse, that having grown used to a teat she might never learn to feed from the breast. I have never felt so sad.

Third day home, I rang a friend of mine in Brisbane, a doctor and a mother of two who had qualified some years before as a lactation consultant. Pam Douglas is a different kind of doctor. She doesn't like much about the medical profession. We had met through her husband,

and at first we did not understand each other. I am the sort of person who says, 'I think ...' She is the sort of person who says, 'I feel ...' But over the years we had come to enjoy the differences between us, and now I wanted her wisdom. Now our roles were reversed. I cried on the telephone to her. 'It's awful, Pam,' I said.

'There is so much I could say to you,' she replied, 'but you need expert help.' Within half an hour, she had found me the name of a lactation consultant near where we live: Cheryl Hanson, of Lithgow. 'Is there such a thing as a lactation consultant?' my father said, bemused, when we told him where we were going. He had already told me my baby was fine, but then my father is a very rational man.

We hit the road, Warwick in his overalls and what I call his dead ferret jumper. I can't remember how I was dressed—certainly not in anything clean.

Meanwhile, in Brisbane, Pam was writing me a letter that she never posted. It was an angry letter. 'What if,' Pam wrote, 'given that her jaundice is mild and became obvious on day three, and given that this kind of jaundice is a common, self-limiting condition, no one had taken her blood? Then no one would have said, "That's higher than expected".' Pam wrote that a baby with significant jaundice is easily detected, that they could have safely waited. Pam said that blood level tests in jaundice correspond with the spread of the yellow colour over the body, so that the levels shown in the test should hardly have been a surprise.

'What if no one said, "She's drowsy because of the jaundice"?' Pam said this kind of jaundice is helped by frequent breastfeeds, but does not cause drowsiness. 'What if she wasn't weighed, since all her behaviour has been to date normal neo-natal behaviour, and she has been reasonably content?' Pam wrote. 'There is no good reason to weigh at that time, since weight loss in the first few days is usual, and what are you going to do about weight loss anyway, other than support breastfeeding? It is far more dangerous to introduce formula, given all that we know now.

'What if all the health professionals around you believed that both you and the baby were absolutely capable of weathering the bumps and irregularities of the first few weeks ... without the threat of major disaster looming? What if they had told you that there was room for bad nights and a run of upsetting feeds ... if this had happened, would you be quite so sleepless, so concerned ... would the nights be riven by the nightmares and the sleeplessness then? Would the terror of your failure, her death, loom out of the shadows?'

While Pam was writing, Warwick and I were talking to Cheryl Hanson. She said: 'Look, I know babies. I am a midwife. This is a healthy baby.' She said: 'I know, in the middle of the night you feel all alone,' and when I broke down in tears, she let me cry. In fact, she had several boxes of tissues at the ready. Then she taught me some things about breastfeeding.

You see, Cheryl was used to seeing mothers in the condition I was in. It is not unusual. The only thing that is more common is for mothers not to call for help, to give up breastfeeding, and to go deeper into the darkness before surfacing. For me, the darkness lifted that day. We learned some new techniques. We went home. I slept, and although it was not all plain sailing from there, things got better. Clare learned to smile, and I like to think she learned it from me.

Last week, I went to see Cheryl again, this time to talk to her about this essay. Unlike all the other interviews I do with important men, this time Clare came too. She smiled at the strangers in the street. She sat in my arms as I carried her, and she looked about. A breastfed baby—nearly three times her birth weight—and all grown by me! Her little head went bob bob, and I thought: what is this love? 'To love' is a verb—a doing word—but loving Clare is not something I do. It is something that I am.

Cheryl Hanson did the lactation consultant's course at her own expense, but she doesn't work in the field. There are no jobs. The local hospital doesn't see the need. 'But who do the midwives ring when they've got real problems?' Cheryl asked Clare, standing her on her knee. (Clare likes being stood on people's knees, needing help only to balance. Whenever she is on her feet she opens her mouth. It is as though her knees were connected to her jaw. Unfold legs. Open mouth.)

'What was your first impression of me?' I asked Cheryl.

'You were physically exhausted, emotionally drained. You obviously didn't care how you looked. I thought you might be a hippy sort of a person. The questions you asked were sensible questions, even though you were upset. And you weren't worried about breastfeeding in front of me. Some mothers won't. That spoke volumes.'

Cheryl told me about a mother who was bottle feeding, but whose baby began to nuzzle her breast one day and feed without encouragement. The woman's husband was furious. 'We only just got your body back,' he said.

'Most women still think bottle feeding is better,' she said.

'Still?' I asked

'Yes. They say you can see how much the baby is getting. It's scientific . . .'

We talked about science.

'I remember my baby sister screaming at the other end of the house for hours on end,' Cheryl said. 'You fed on schedule, and you put the baby down. That was how it was done. If you did that, you were a good mother.'

These days, though, the advice has changed. My baby care book advocates 'attachment parenting'. Never leave your baby to cry. Take your baby to bed with you. Carry your baby in a sling wherever you go.

This book, and several others, state without qualification that scientific studies have proved that the more you carry a baby, the less it cries. Some weeks ago, I went looking for the original studies on which this advice was based, and of course the picture wasn't as simple as the baby books would have you believe. Propaganda cannot admit complexity or ambiguity.

In 1986, Doctors Hunziker and Barr at the McGill University in Montreal studied 99 mother-infant pairs. Half were assigned to carry their infants through the day, and the others were a control group. The carried infants cried and fussed 41 per cent less overall and 51 per cent less during the evening hours. This is the study those who would have mothers carry babies choose to quote.

But in 1993, researchers, including some of those involved in the original study, published another piece of research. They had studied 38 mother-infant pairs where the infant had been diagnosed as having colic. (The medical definition of colic is crying for more than three hours a day every day for at least one week. Cheryl Hanson's comment: 'I don't believe in colic.')

The researchers assigned different groups different methods of treatment—extra carrying, the use of a device that simulated the movement of a car, and a control group that was only counselled. The researchers expected to find that carrying decreased the crying, but instead they discovered no significant differences between the groups. Yet another study looked at 66 mother-infant pairs with colic. Again, they found that extra carrying made no difference.

Publishing their findings, the researchers speculated whether the differences in the results were because it was too late to intervene once 'colic' was established, or whether there was some problem with the sample. None of these ambiguities are reflected in the advice given to mothers. The baby books are quite certain about what sort of creatures children are, and what sort of people mothers should be.

The Baby Book by William and Martha Sears, which contains all sorts of useful advice, and on which I have often depended, is quite clear in its political message. The attachment parented children they know have grown up to be 'bothered by social injustices and [they] do something to correct them. These kids cared! Because they were so firmly rooted in their inner sensitivity, they were willing to swim upstream against the current. These children will become the movers and shakers and leaders and shapers of a better world to come.'

'If you are going to buy a child care book, only buy one,' Cheryl Hanson told me the first morning I met her, but I didn't take her advice. I read them all. Old ones, and new ones.

At the beginning of this century, motherhood became scientific. The paediatrician Luther Holt was opposed to the 'promiscuous' kissing of babies, lest it spread infection. The most important thing in rearing, he said, was regularity. Playing with young babies, making them laugh, imposed a dangerous strain on their nervous system.

Next was John B. Watson, a behavioural psychologist who published *The Psychological Care of Infant and Child* in 1928, in which he fulminated against cuddling and affection for fear of spoiling the child. To pick up a child between feeds was to invite moral laxity. Toilet training was to begin at one month. Watson brought up two boys of his own by his principles, never betraying any affection for either of them, although their mother apparently managed to sneak in a cuddle now and then. The boys grew up into sane adults, which only proves how robust children can be.

These authors, too, were quite certain that the children raised by their methods would be the shapers of a better world to come.

By these standards, the famous Dr Spock was permissive. So permissive, in fact, that in one of the most obvious connections between baby rearing advice and politics, he was explicitly blamed for the student riots in the 1960s. His advice, it was said, had created a generation of layabouts who knew no discipline. Now, of course, those layabouts are parents, and reading new advice books.

In the shift from Spock to the full blown 'trust your instincts' approach, one book is a fundamental part of the shift from the faith in science through the 50s and 60s, to the romanticising of the 'natural' in the 70s. It is *The Continuum Concept* by Jean Liedloff, first published in 1975 and cited in the bibliography of just about every baby book since (or at least, those that have bibliographies).

Liedloff lived among the Yequana Indians in deepest South America. The Yequana were still living their traditional lifestyle. Their world, Liedloff said, was an idyll. The Yequana knew no unhappiness. They had no word for 'work' because all of life was play.

'They were the happiest people I had seen anywhere,' she wrote. 'I seldom had a clear sense that they were of the same species as ourselves, though of course if asked I should have said so without hesitation. The children were uniformly well behaved, they never fought, were never punished, always obeyed happily and instantly.'

Liedloff argued passionately that the Yequana's ways were more 'correct' than ours because they had an unbroken continuum with evolution. They were human beings living in their natural habitat. 'Civilised' people, on the other hand, had strayed too far from the continuum. Liedloff attributed virtually all of western civilisation's ills to the fact that infants were left to cry alone, rather than being carried around next to their mothers.

Among the Yequana, babies were carried all day long and lay down with their mothers to sleep at night. Child care was regarded as 'nothing to do'. Babies simply accompanied their mothers as they worked. Nor were parents protective. Babies were left to play with knives, with fire, and near dangerous falls. They were trusted to look after themselves, and according to Liedloff, accidents were rare.

When accidents did happen, the parents were relatively unconcerned. Liedloff tells of treating one little boy shot with an arrow by his brother. The mother looked in, saw the horrific wound, but when she saw her son was being looked after, she walked away. 'There was no need for her to stay . . . his mother assumed that if he needed her, he would come to her, and she was available for any such eventuality.'

Liedloff contrasts tribal life with a harrowing account of the feelings of a typical western baby, left to cry in his cot:

The infant's waking hours are passed in yearning, waiting on interminable waiting for rightness to replace the silent void. For a few minutes a day his longing is suspended and his terrible skin crawling need to be touched, to be held and moved about, is relieved . . . at first it is hard for her to put him down after feeding, especially because he cries so desperately when she does. But she is convinced that she must, for her mother has told her that if she gives in to him now, he will be spoiled and cause trouble later. She wants to do everything right . . . softly she closes the door. She has declared war upon him. Her will must prevail over his. Through the door she hears what sounds like someone being tortured. Her continuum sense recognises it as such. Nature does not make clear signals that someone is being tortured unless it is the case. IT IS PRECISELY AS SERIOUS AS IT SOUNDS . . . (Liedloff's emphasis)

* * *

Clare and I have just been to hang out the nappies. The sun is out, but the air is cool. I worry about whether she is dressed warmly enough. She sits on my hip in the sling. Clare likes the sling. She has sat on my hip at airports, meetings, and while I work, but when I write she prefers the floor, or to be with her father. Writing is boring for a baby. It makes her cry. But I am a writer. I am not a farmer, nor a hunter-gatherer.

Out there by the washing line, my slideshow mind was at work again. I have read something that gave me a similar feel to *The Continuum Concept*—something similar in its ideal vision, and its criticism of the way we live. Something that had nothing to do with motherhood.

Then, click, the slide is on the projector, and I know what I am thinking of. It is the fourth voyage in *Gulliver's Travels*—not the voyages to Lilliput and Brobdingnag that have been popularised in Disney-style cartoons, but the dark, disturbing journey to a land governed by wonderful, intelligent talking horses, who call themselves Houyhnhnms.

The Houyhnhnms knew no unhappiness. They had no word for 'lie', because it was not conceivable to them that they would say 'the thing that is not'. They had no need for politics, since it was always perfectly clear to them what should be done, and there was no dissent. They had difficulty understanding the word 'opinion'. Death accepted without remorse. One Houyhnhnm used the death of her husband as an excuse for being late for a lunch appointment. She showed no sadness. Marriage was decided on purely rational grounds. There was no love, and no anger.

Gulliver worshipped them, but there was a worm in the apple. The land of the Houyhnhnms was inhabited by another species, the Yahoos—bestial, unteachable, ugly brutes, always fighting and fornicating and kept in kennels by the Houyhnhnms. Gulliver said, 'As to those filthy Yahoos . . . I confess I never saw any sensitive Being so detestable on all Accounts, and the more I came near them, the more hateful they grew.'

The problem is, the Houyhnhnms think Gulliver is a Yahoo, and he is slowly forced to realise that the Yahoos are indeed human beings. Gulliver hates the Yahoos, which means he hates himself. He tries to become as much like a Houyhnhnm as possible. He flinches when he catches sight of his Yahoo-face in a mirror. He doesn't hesitate to replace his clothes, when they wear out, with ones made from Yahoo skin. Forced to return to his own society, he cannot bear to have his wife or children near him.

When *Gulliver's Travels* was first published, Swift was castigated for the fourth voyage. He was interpreted as displaying an unremitting hatred of humanity. More modern criticism has suggested that Gulliver was wrong when he concluded that humanity and the Yahoos were one and the same. The Houyhnhnms, these critics suggested, represented Plato's ideal of a society based entirely on reason. The Yahoos represented Hobbes's view of humanity as a brutal, animalistic existence.

Neither of these two extremes were humanity. Instead Gulliver himself, part rational being and part animal, represented what it was to be human, and he was a tragic figure because of his inability to accept that this imperfect mix was his nature. Perhaps, the critics suggested, there was something chilly, something even slightly ridiculous, in the perfection of the Houyhnhnms. Perhaps their ideal was not so admirable. Perhaps we needed our human affections, our passions.

Liedloff reminds me of Gulliver. Both are travellers, both are enamoured by what they find, and both are disgusted and dismayed when they return to their own societies.

The irony is that, whereas Gulliver worshipped a society based on reason, and saw the Yahoos as repugnant because they were animals, Liedloff believes the ideal lies in our animal nature, and that it is reason that should be distrusted. 'Ever more frequently our innate sense of what is best for us is short circuited by suspicion, while the intellect, which has never known much about our real needs, decides what to do. It is not ... the province of the reasoning faculty to decide how a baby ought to be treated,' she writes.

Liedloff, of course, was reporting facts, and Gulliver and the Houyhnhnms were fiction, but now I will be picky. Liedloff says that the Yequana babies never cry, yet elsewhere she writes that on the rare occasions when they do cry, mothers hiss in their ears to quiet them. I look in the index. There are many references to crying. All are to western babies. None of the mentions of the Yequana babies' crying are indexed.

Liedloff says the Yequana know no unhappiness, yet the tribal leader tries to stop Liedloff leaving, because her medical skills have become so valuable to the tribe. He is prepared to risk one of his men dying rather than allow Liedloff to leave, and take him with her to hospital.

Sometimes travellers see what they want to see, and sometimes what they see is a mould of their own preoccupations.

* * *

Perhaps Liedloff would say my very intellectualising of this debate, my examination of her index, my desk covered with scientific papers and literary criticism, are part of the problem. When rationality is denied, there are no grounds from which one can argue. One can only feel.

So here I sit, strung between the babbling voice on the floor by my feet, and my intellect. Here I sit, breastfeeding from my office chair, leafing through the papers on my desk, being suspicious of what books tell me, looking back to the original research. Thinking, writing, changing nappies, feeling the tug of my heart and the workings of my mind. Neither animal nor entirely rational creature.

Now Clare has gone out with her father so I can finish this article, and I am missing her little warm head, and her little hands, and the sound of her voice. They will be home soon, and I am nearly finished.

We will have lunch together. She will eat her little scraps of mashed pumpkin and mashed banana. The tablecloth will not be as clean as it should be. Warwick and I will not make particularly profound conversation. This essay is not as perfect as it should be.

Later, Clare will fall asleep in our bed. Dear little animal. Next to me I will feel the length of her, the width of her, the reality of her. Her eyes will be fixed on mine while she sucks on the breast. Then she will drop off to sleep.

She is neither Yahoo nor Houyhnhnm nor Yequana. I will not have her serve as the mirror for other people, for their ideas of what we all should be.

Clare is herself, here and now, and the middle is quite possibly the right place to be.

* * *

References:

Ronald G. Barr and others, 'Carrying as Colic "Therapy": A Randomised Controlled Trial' *Pediatrics* 87: 5 May 1991.

Ivor H. Evans (ed), *Brewer's Dictionary of Phrase and Fable* Cassell: 1983.

Robert A. Greenberg (ed), *Swift's 'Gulliver's Travels'*, *a Norton Critical Edition* Norton: 1970.

Urs A. Hunziker MD and Ronald G. Barr MDCM, FRCP, 'Increased Carrying Reduces Infant Crying: A Randomised Controlled Trial' *Pediatrics* 77: 5 May 1986.

Jean Liedloff, *The Continuum Concept* Duckworth: 1975 (reprinted Penguin Arkana).

Ian St James Roberts PhD and others, 'Supplementary Carrying Compared with Advice to Increase Responsive Parenting as Interventions to Prevent Persistent Infant Crying' *Pediatrics* 95: 3 March 1995.

William and Martha Sears, *The Baby Book—Everything You Need to Know about Your Baby from Birth to Age Two* Little, Brown & Company: 1993.

Shari L. Thurer, *The Myths of Motherhood: How Culture Reinvents the Good Mother* Penguin: 1994.

John B. Watson, *The Psychological Care of Infant and Child* W. Norton & Co: 1928.

JILL SINGER
The Shadow Behind Me

When a schoolmate discovered how babies 'got in there' she nearly threw up, and vowed to anyone who'd listen that she'd insist on anaesthesia before any future husband could impregnate her. It made good sense at the time. Better still, we'd all remain spinsters and forget about having kids. Learning about all the starving babies in Africa cemented our resolve. Breeding was irresponsible as well as very rude. Keep in mind here we were pre-pubescent, our full complement of hormones hadn't yet kicked in.

But what I really don't understand, now I'm a grown-up, is how people can still ask you to justify your decision to have a child. What on earth do they expect you to say? Oh well, the truth is I was sick of having a social life? My body was looking a little too taut and I thought

I should wreck it? My career was cruising along nicely and I'm terrified of success? It's a question only mothers and fathers of none ask. Like the former schoolmate who viewed the fruit of my womb with disdain and then pronounced she'd had a 'tubal litigation'. Thank Freud that genetic material was nipped in the bud.

Deliberate non-parents can be very smug. They know they can dip into their cosmetics purse and confidently extract an intact lipstick. They know the image of their BMW won't be sullied by a vomit-stained booster seat strapped in the back. They know their breasts will stay perky for just that little bit longer. I say 'little bit' because I have a theory about this body stuff. Many women spend a lot of time trying to stave off the ravages of time, defying mortality and mourning their spent youth—a perfectly legitimate way to spend time of course. But the suggestion that child-bearing ruins a woman's body is a furphy. It's gravity that gets you in the end. If you line up a whole lot of elderly women I'll bet it's impossible to pick which ones have had children and which haven't. When it's all said and done, we all sag and wrinkle to much the same extent. I mean, how many perky octogenarian breasts have you seen lately? And really, if they *were* perky, how sad if it came at the cost of not being able to spruik about young Jason and Kylie, and how well they're doing at school, and how everyone says they're just like you and have your eyes, you know, before they started to crêpe and droop around the edges . . .

I find it difficult to talk about how intensely happy (and occasionally suicidal) having a child has made me. I recall a drunken conversation back in second-year uni. The topic was what rooted us to the earth. For Anne, it was God. She seemed so sure of this, and I envied her that elusive thing called faith. For Paul, it was Art. This seemed slightly more understandable but still a little airy-fairy and unconvincing (but much admired by the others). I blush to confess I couldn't think of what rooted me to the earth. This admission provoked considerable vilification. It was construed as shallowness—an unpardonable sin. Years later my daughter gazed into my eyes as she was sucking at my breast, one tiny hand patting at the free nipple. She would break her suction now and then to have a chortle. My insides lurched like when you fancy the cut of a bloke's jib, only better. I was well and truly rooted.

There are inherent problems in rooting oneself to the earth through a child. What happens if the child comes to loathe you, is stolen, or should die? My God, what happens if everything should go well and it smilingly leaves you one day for A Life Of Its Own? Others have provided wise counsel in this area. For example, the experience of my friends Jack and Lina whose first child was born deformed and extremely sick. Being a doctor, Jack realised immediately that Anne was not long for this world. The fashion then in such circumstances was to leave the child in the draught of an open window and hardly feed it. It took Anne 18 days to die—agony for her and hell for her parents. Many years later, Lina says if it happened again, she'd take the baby home and nurture it until it died, even if it prolonged the dying. What struck me most about their story was the grim humour with which they told it, and their ability to get on with life. Because of his professional status, Jack was allowed to collect Anne's body. The couple gently placed her in a shoe box and stepped into the hospital lift where another couple was on its way to the labour ward, the woman clearly well into labour. 'Shall we lift the lid?' Lina whispered into Jack's ear. They cracked up laughing at their own macabre awfulness. Subsequently they got on their bikes and rode around Europe, came home, and had three sons.

I've spoken with many parents who have suffered the agony of losing a child. The thought of it has haunted me from the moment my daughter was born. Since I lacked any religious faith, it was this little shadow trotting behind me who miraculously cast the light in front. When she was tiny, a childhood dream returned to me, with a twist—whenever I was chased by bogey-men I could always escape by flying. No wings were involved, just an extremely vigorous arm flapping motion. A reliable launching place was from the sundeck of my family home. Take-off was the hardest part, and the bad men would get very close to nabbing me by the toes before I got up sufficient momentum. Then along came the nipper. She would cling to me like a little monkey as I leaped forward across the valley and flew toward Mount Donna Buang. The additional flapping required, and consequent arm strain, was considerable. My waking hours became plagued by tendonitis in my shoulders. To this very day, my shoulders seize up at the first sign of stress.

Now the nipper's as big as me and comes out with stuff like: 'You've got to learn to let go', 'You're too smothering'—or worse—'You're neurotic'. She has a point. The thing is, I refuse to relax until I know she's independently flapping along beside me on my nocturnal flights. Surely most mothers feel like this? When pressed, the ones I know confess to it. The hypothetical question, 'How would you cope if your child died?' is usually answered with, 'Immediate suicide' (unless they have more than one child, then it is realised that any right to a quick exit has been foregone). A close friend has only changed her response to this after several months on Prozac.

Another mate, Sue, was horrified during a recent plane flight. It was a rough journey, the plane lurching up and down alarmingly. What disturbed Sue most was that her fear was for herself, and not for the daughter sitting beside her. When it came to the crunch she was a bad mother. We did consider the possibility that her reaction was an indication of mental wellness but, you know, the guilt lingers. This is what happens when you become a mother. It's a constant bloody worry.

Then there's the blowhole down the Victorian coast. Large expanses of angry water and children are a terrifying combination. Kiddies just love looking down the blowhole. Mothers tend to screech, 'Not too close!' when the kiddies are a) still 10 metres from the fenced edge, and b) 19 years old. Lina (mother of three, you remember, lost the first) is so together she even knows how to cope with the blowhole. I swore that if *my* nipper fell in, I'd feel compelled to jump in after her, even in the full knowledge we would both surely perish. But Lina, she's smart. She'd look around first to see if any bloke was preparing himself to jump in after her kid. If not, *then* she'd go in. That woman has been a big help.

Which brings me to men.

Before I continue I'll give the usual disclaimer. Some of my closest friends are men, and they're utterly delightful human beings. Some of them are even fathers, and have warmed to the task admirably. That said, I am of the opinion that single fathers have a much easier go of it than single mothers. Women—oestrogen seeping out of their every pore—flock around them wanting to help. Men who turn up to work with a kiddie can fully expect it to be cheerfully passed around the office and universally praised. Women who pull this stunt are seen as professionally messy. Mind you, I'm not outraged by this, merely jealous. It's not as though there are any reciprocal trade-offs. Any useful atavistic male urges don't seem to emerge at the sight of a single mother. Men don't start manically hunting and gathering or strutting around in search of leaking taps, wielding a spanner and such like. Oh no. They want her to hire a handyman as well as a babysitter, and quit the whingeing.

And another thing. We've all worked with women who say they can't come along to staff meetings, social functions, etc, because of family commitments. What you never hear is women referring to this as 'babysitting'. Some blokes do. 'Babysitting' their own kids ... and then they get shitty if things bugger up and the Family Court doesn't give them the custodial first prize. Well knock me over with a feather, sunshine.

The nipper reckons I'm too hard on blokes. She says it's a generational thing and that my mates and I are tragic, but she still gets a good laugh out of us.

Most of the women I know (and the odd bloke) worry that our children haven't been given a good grounding in sustainable coupling. How to play Happy Families. How to be Normal. (As I said, maternal guilt is all pervasive.) Bettina Arndt is no help. Many a pinot has been hurled down the gullet while we wonder what to do about Bettina. You see, apparently Bettina bagged herself a rich hubby and they had a little one together. Good on them, I say. Bettina adds to the material comfort of their nest by writing newspaper articles in which she claims things like this: 'In choosing to raise children in a single parent family, the sad truth is many [women] are sentencing them to a lesser life ... the huge increase in single mothers is occurring in the face of growing evidence of potential risks to children of being raised by a sole parent.'

What these bad mothers are doing, according to Bettina, is raising their children in poverty (how bloody selfish can you get?). Almost half of single mothers, she says, are on pensions (I wonder how many men don't cough up their child support?). To make matters worse, Bettina quotes a Western Australian study which indicates that children of single parent families face more than twice the risk of mental health problems compared with those who live with both parents. (I mean, they can't be screwed up because of anything Dad did, could they? And does 'facing the risk' mean they actually *have* a problem, or that their environment offends certain standards of normality?)

And there's more. Bettina says single mothers can't expect to improve their lot by wedding some bloke who didn't sire their nipper: 'Many of these women may eventually marry, but generally this does not improve the outcomes for their children ... children in step-families also show more emotional problems ...'

By the time I had read most of Bettina's article I was ready to cut either my wrists or her throat. So many rules to follow in order to be a good mother, and I had broken them all.

Now don't get me wrong. I'm very happy for Bettina that her legally wed partner is well-off and presumably not prone to hitting the sauce and belting her up. And if he ever does tire of her and nick off with some little missy, I will strenuously fight any feeling of *schadenfreude*.

The nipper has just read this and told me to calm down. 'The woman is just a drop-kick,' she reckons. I wish you could see the nipper. Does anecdotal evidence count? She's witty, smart, funny. My pride and joy. No sign of a facial tic. She's managing to glide through adolescence with considerable dignity. She hasn't yet to my knowledge burned down a single hedge.

'Darling,' I said. 'Darling, we have to be vigilant about this stuff. It's nasty politics at work.' Then I gave her a copy of a speech to read—'The Bankruptcy of Conservative Political Ideas' by the Evatt Foundation's former director Dr Peter Botsman. In it, he focuses on the New Right's allegations that there's a glut of single young women in the United States who are deliberately getting pregnant to go on welfare—a myth propagated here as well as there by those who want to cut welfare payments. The fact is, while the proportion of births to poor, black single mothers has grown in America in the past 30 years, this is because middle-class and affluent blacks are choosing to have fewer children in wedlock, not because the poor women are rushing to breed more than they did in the past. I'm sure the same is done with statistics here. Wealthy, white, wedded women and their chums can harp on all they like about welfare and single mothers, but the fact remains, the materially luckier women don't tend to breed a lot.

In any case, no matter how much financial or marital

security people might think they have, you can still always find someone who'll rabbit on about the 'right time' to have a child. Save up, get hitched, pay off the car and the house, put away money for the school fees, squeeze in a spot of travel, get that promotion. They're scared, I reckon—trying to insulate themselves from the terrifying insecurity that parenthood brings.

I'm here to tell you that's impossible. Having a child is like a leap of faith. You jump, and then somehow all the pain and the joy of being alive starts to make sense.

JENNY TABAKOFF
Bed

There is that familiar noise again. A thud, followed by 10 footsteps, then another, softer, thud right next to you.

'Mummy?'

No reply. To start up a conversation at this time of night is fatal.

'Mummy.'

No reply again.

'Love you, Mummy.'

You relent. 'Love you, little man.'

The little bundle next to you sighs, curls up contentedly and is instantly asleep again. You cannot help but admire, even in the dark, the soft, rounded arms and cheeks, and wonder again at the elegance which comes so easily, so naturally to the very young in sleep.

You wake up the following morning with a cricked neck and the feeling that someone's feet are in your face. That is because they are.

* * *

When our first son was born we stood firm. We'd had, after all, some inkling that our bed might be under threat.

'Don't *ever* let them come into bed with you,' experienced parents had said within minutes of discovering that I was pregnant. 'There has to be *somewhere* in your life that is sacred, somewhere that is child-free.'

They had said other things, too, of course, but sleep was the issue uppermost in every parent's mind. Inevitably their parting words would be: 'Get all the sleep you can now, because once you have kids your sleep will never be the same again.'

I absorbed the message that interrupted sleep would become part of the pattern of our lives. But what I had never appreciated, and what people never tell you, is how babies change your relationship with your bed. Friends say, and books confirm, that your sex life might never be the same, or your body, or your relationship with your own mother. But they never say that your bed—the place where parenthood generally begins—will become a combination of playground, battlefield, stage, trampoline and crèche. They never tell you that children will raid it, jump on it, throw up in it, wet it, and even bleed on it. They never warn that one day you might need to wear crampons to bed just to have a chance of clinging on to the edge of the mattress.

Still, we had some sense of foreboding, and for many months after our first child was born, our bed remained our own. Of course, we never slept the same again. That blissful, selfish slumber of old vanished the night we brought him home from hospital. Night feeds seemed to go on interminably, the next one seeming to start as soon as the last had finished. Other people's babies slept three, four, eight hours between feeds, but ours never did.

The baby spent his first months in a bassinet at the end of our bed and when he woke, ravenous, I resolutely sat in an antique nursing chair to feed him. No way were we going to allow him to invade our bed. I would look out the window at the two am inner-city goings-on: the van which would unload its cargo in the night, its driver and passenger furtively looking around; the drunks swaying down the footpath; the warring husband and wife a few doors down having yet another domestic; the ancient rustbucket cars that roared down the street, mufflers shattered and stereos booming.

Amongst the exhaustion of interrupted sleep and whirring hormones, I had strange hallucinations: in one dream I heard the baby crying yet again. My dream self rushed up the stairs and found my baby waiting for me at the top, transformed into a fully-grown adult.

That did it. After that night, when he awoke, I would pick him up and go back to bed, lying on one side while he quietly and contentedly suckled. Sometimes I fell asleep before him and he stayed there all night. Sometimes he fell asleep before me and I would reach into one of those old reserves of heartlessness and put him back in his bassinet. But the fortress had been breached: our bed was never quite our own again.

Despite our constant fears, we never accidentally rolled on him. Somehow even a few kilograms of humanity is able to establish its own space—rather a lot of it, in fact. We often found ourselves crammed into one corner of the bed while our infant son spread himself out luxuriantly over acres of mattress. Of course we should have moved him, if not back to his bassinet then at least to a more reasonable amount of our territory. But this small scrap of humanity had outmanoeuvred us: if we moved him he might wake, if he woke he would cry, and if he cried we might never get back to sleep. And sleep was everything to us, something of which he was well aware. There could be no other explanation for the absolute confidence of his sleeping position: arms up and out, legs all over the place—but most often in our stomachs.

The baby moved from a bassinet to a cot in his own

bedroom. The night feeds miraculously came to an end and then came the happy morning when I realised that he had not woken at all. But even when he 'slept through' regularly, I never did again. My sleep was shallower, more fitful. That old umbilical link seemed to remain, and my eyes would open at any rustle from the cot—and if there was no noise, that was even more worrying. Those preaching parents had been right about one thing after all.

In the mornings, we would pick him up and spend a happy 10 minutes with him in our bed, trying to detect the beginnings of speech in his gurgling noises, watching the fleeting expressions of dead relatives flit across his face, listening to his delighted giggles as we pulled faces, or played peekaboo, or tickled his tummy.

Pretty soon he got the impression that our bed was his bed, and there was nowhere in the world he would rather be.

* * *

The toys began their inexorable march across the house. One rattle multiplied into huge plastic constructions and mountains of teddies and rabbits which took over the bedroom, the living room, the house. Our son grew too long for his cot, and agile enough to hop out when he got restless. It was time to buy him a bed.

This confirmed his own impression that he was a big boy, and he happily oversaw the dismantling of the cot. But that evening he said: 'I want to sleep in your bed.'

We were firm. 'This is your bed now,' we said, pointing at his narrow mattress. There ensued a struggle that went on for several weeks, punctuated by many unnecessary visits to the bathroom, many requests for milk that went undrunk. To make it seem a friendlier place, we took to lying down with him and having a five-minute chat about this and that (what happened that day, how steam trains worked, why the dinosaurs died out), followed by a little sing-song in which 'Daisy, Daisy', 'Tipperary' and the entire Al Jolson canon figured prominently. Then, 'Night night, sleep tight, don't wake up till the morning light', we would say, more in hope than expectation, and he would fall asleep in his bed quite happily.

But the rules always changed long before the morning light—usually around two am, in fact. If he fell out of bed, or woke up needing a drink or a wee, the same request always went up: 'I want to sleep in your bed.'

It is hard for a mother to argue in the middle of the night.

'Why?' you ask irritably.

'Because I love you.'

Your resolve melts: how can you say no to this gorgeous little person to whom you mean everything? How many people are there in this life to whom your very presence, just your smell and proximity, can bring such complete and innocent happiness?

'All right,' you say. 'Just this once.'

* * *

The labour pains began around six pm on a Sunday. This birth was much quicker and less painful than the first, and within a couple of hours Stuart and I were gazing at each other over the suckling form of our second son. I had a sleepless night in hospital, vainly trying to stifle my excitement, gazing with wonder at this tiny form with its scrawny legs and tight-fisted grip, and attempting to figure out which grandparent he took after.

My husband and older son picked me up from hospital the following morning. The house we had left only yesterday as a family of three we now re-entered as a family of four. I was hungry, sore, relieved, grateful and exhausted, but this was one of those occasions when these five adjectives added up to just one word: ecstatic.

We sat there, all of us stunned in our various ways, ate ham sandwiches and pondered what we would do with the rest of this special day. 'Let's have a sleep,' I said, and we climbed the stairs and lay down together: Stuart, Oscar, Nathan and I.

There was lots of room in our bed that first time. We

slept for hours. How can I describe the strange wonder of sleeping all together, in the middle of a working day? A sleep that to this day seemed more significant than a mere nap, because it somehow knitted us together in the mysterious fabric that is a family?

The baby whimpered. I gave him a sleepy feed lying down. He slept on. The rest of us gazed and laughed at his tiny fingers, his puzzled, windy frowns, his exclamations at the rumbles in his gut. And then we, too, slept on.

The hours passed: warm, cuddling, happy hours. If we woke, it was only to commit another feature, another expression, another fingernail to memory, or to wonder at how passing wind made him look like great uncle Wally. Some things remained unsaid, because how could anyone find the words to describe the sight of this tiny new form sleeping on the bed in which he had been conceived?

And then it was over. We woke, bathed, had a cup of tea, and normal life resumed. The next day Stuart went back to work, Oscar went back to pre-school, and I began the process of showing the new baby off to friends and family, and selfconsciously taking him shopping for the first time.

* * *

Somehow the double bed, which had once been big enough only for two, then three, was suddenly big enough for four—just as our family had mysteriously expanded to encompass this new baby, even though we had never imagined we could love another child as we loved our first.

The baby would go to sleep in his bassinet or cot, but when he woke for a feed we just pulled him into bed with us and he either stayed or left depending on circumstances, sleepiness or parental resolve. In the mornings, and sometimes in the middle of the night, his big brother would pad in and join us. We got used to that sound: thud, 10 little steps, thud again, and then, 'Mummy, I want to lie with you'.

Of course, it was never as perfect as it had been that first day. 'Stop kicking,' we would say. 'Stop talking.' Or: 'Look, if you can't lie still . . .'

Sometimes it was too hot, or so cold that the battle for the doona made life impossible and one of the adults would crack and stalk off to the children's room. Sometimes the baby would want to stick his fingers up our noses or in our ears just to see what was in there. Sometimes he would vomit, or someone would have an accident or a nosebleed, and we would have to throw everyone out to change the sheets. Sometimes we just wanted a good night's sleep and determinedly carried each intruder back to his own bed.

But enough of that initial contentment remained. Even now, when both boys have beds of their own, they often wake up with us. They can find their way in pitch dark, in strange hotels, over any obstacle. They never trip, fall or bump into door frames. It is the kind of homing instinct worthy of scientific study.

It is all very different from my own childhood, when my parents' bedroom was a sanctuary with an invisible but unmistakable 'Do Not Disturb' sign on the door. It could never be entered except after a discreet knock, and only with a very good excuse. I was only allowed to disturb its pale lilac privacy with a duster in one hand, while doing my round of Saturday morning chores.

Certainly I can never remember crawling over my mother's face the way that my sons crawl over mine, or lying in bed to have a chat with her about this and that. To many people, this generational change might be evidence of declining standards of parenting, but now I cannot imagine life any other way.

Usually no word is spoken. There is just the sound of footsteps followed by a soft thud in the bed beside you. Often the boys arrive within minutes of each other. Occasionally they have had a nightmare. Sometimes they are feverish, or unwell, or sad, or cuddly, or frightened of the dark. Whatever the problem, lying in the big bed is the answer, the medicine, the consolation.

Sometimes we complain of cricked necks, and grumble about kicking and doona-hogging. But often we never even know that one of them has found his way to us, and only realise when a plump arm is thrown carelessly in our faces, or the clock radio goes off and we see an immobile lump under the doona beside us.

Things go rapidly downhill from there. Any morning lying-in session invariably ends in disarray. The little one does indeed say, 'Roll over', just like in the song. This is followed by some hilarity (not to say hysteria) as the two boys wriggle backwards down the bed, or have a leg wrestle that ends in a fight, or decide they want to jump up and down. Memories of sleeping in and breakfast in bed are as distant and mythical to us as King Arthur or Robin Hood.

If we mention any of this to other parents, they still say: 'Why do you let them come into your bed? Didn't anyone tell you? You must have been crazy.'

And yet, and yet . . . How to explain that it still seems a wonderfully happy thing, this padding of feet, the reassurance you can give just by being there, those occasional moments of peace and contentment that stir memories of the first time your family all slept together? And that it is all the more wonderful because you know that one day soon it will all end, that your children will no longer want to crawl into bed with you and just snuggle up?

Bed used to be your own personal playground, belonging to just the two of you—now you share it with someone else. How to explain that when you become parents, what happens to your bed seems somehow resonant of something bigger? That it can expand just as your life can, and that there is always room for one more.

And that is OK. More than that, it is absolutely right.

PENNY BIGGINS
Nature's Quirky Little Ways

I had always assumed that conceiving a child would be as easy and uneventful as deciding whether to have chops or steak for dinner, and I suspect we often put more thought into the latter. After all, it is said that our bodies are designed to reproduce, if nothing else, though should I ever meet the designer I'll have a few words to say to him, her or it.

When I turned 30 I noticed that family, friends and the butcher no longer seemed terribly interested in my opinions on such things as nuclear disarmament or whether I wanted chops or steak for dinner, but were only concerned as to When We Were Going To Start Our Family.

'We're starting it now,' we casually and foolishly announced one day and were a little surprised when six months later we hadn't.

Our GP reassured us that this was quite normal and advised us to come back six months later if nothing happened. Nothing did.

At this stage I wasn't unduly alarmed as my menstrual cycle had never been particularly regular. I've always been impressed with women who know that their periods will start at six-and-a-half minutes past five on the third Wednesday of every month. Even now I still get a little surprise when my periods suddenly appear.

We returned from the GP laden down with enough graph paper to chart the current account deficit for the next 50 years and an ovulation thermometer. The purpose of this no-tech equipment is to take your temperature before you get up in the morning and record it on the graph paper. Can there be a more excruciating agony than lying in bed with a thermometer thrust up your private parts when you're desperate to go to the loo? Still, we kept our charts diligently and every time my temperature went up, so did my husband.

It soon became apparent that our child was not, if ever, going to be conceived during a night of passion and all-consuming love because it was during this time that we became overly familiar with the Workman-like Performance. If you're a stranger to this phenomenon it goes like this:

You: 'No, don't go to sleep yet. You can't.'

Him: 'But I'm tired. I've had a really long day.'

You: 'So have I, but we can't go to sleep yet. The chart says we have to do it tonight.'

Him: 'Do we have to? I just don't feel like it.'

You: 'But the chart says . . . '

Him: (tersely) 'Bugger the chart. What's wrong with tomorrow?'

You: (tearfully) 'It'll be too late then. Don't you want a baby?'

Him: 'Not this minute, frankly.'

You: (trying to do something vaguely erotic) 'Oh, go on, it won't take long.'

And it never did.

Yet despite our chart-taking and assiduous workman-like performances, still nothing happened so we upped the ante in the medical stakes and visited a specialist.

And so began our investigation into infertility.

It's easier and cheaper to test the male first and my husband was relieved to discover that he wasn't firing blanks. It was likely then that the problem lay with the target.

At no time did my husband ever make me feel that it was 'my fault' but by now I was starting to feel both baffled and anxious. I was only moderately fit, it must be said, but I was healthy and I wanted a child. Why was my body betraying me like this? Why wouldn't it do what everyone else's did? Women throughout the centuries have spent vast amounts of time and money trying not to get pregnant or going through the traumas of termination. Why was I in the position where the reverse was true?

Mind you, I was cheerfully confident that contemporary medicine could quickly and easily determine what was wrong and fix it.

Back to the specialist.

Maybe he was tired. Perhaps he'd been going through a few workman-like performances of his own, but on all the occasions we saw him, his general manner was one of indifference and remoteness. At least he didn't refer me to a psychiatrist, as another specialist had done to a friend—who only discovered some time later that she had severe endometriosis.

'Right,' said our specialist after briefly gazing at our boxloads of charts. 'Laparoscopy.'

'Which is what exactly?' we enquired deferentially as one does to specialists.

'Under a mild anaesthetic, we insert a small camera through the abdomen ... '

'Ah, womb cam,' I said. The specialist ignored me.

' ... inflate the uterine cavity with carbon dioxide and determine whether the fallopian tubes are patent ... '

'Patent? So seventies!' I said.

I think he'd heard it once or a thousand times before. He ignored me again.

'We also look for any other indications of physiological damage such as endometriosis. See the receptionist and she'll book you in for next week.'

Patient dismissed.

The laparoscopy, which was a painless experience as I was under a general anaesthetic, revealed some very slight endometriosis but the specialist had been unable to determine whether or not my fallopian tubes were patent, which basically means working.

What is it about doctors that they love to play It Pays To Increase Your Word Power with you?

'Hysterosalpingogram.'

'Sorry?' we asked.

'The neck of the cervix is opened, a cannula inserted and dye is injected into the fallopian tubes.'

'Oh?' I started to leave the room. 'Yes, well, I've always thought there are far too many children in the world.'

'See the receptionist and she'll book you in.'

Two weeks later I was lying on a large table, trying to keep perfectly still as instructed while a pair of long-nosed pliers grabbed the neck of my cervix, a length of metal tubing was shoved in and dye was squirted up it. This time there was no anaesthetic.

'It doesn't matter if those bloody tubes are patent or not,' I told my husband. 'I'm unlikely to have sex ever again. Those pliers have finished me off forever.'

He just looked curiously relieved.

Of course, having so publicly declared, now two years before, that we were Starting Our Family, we were inundated with advice from friends and family as to what we should be doing. At first, I didn't really mind because I knew they were just trying to be helpful.

'Go on a holiday, that always works. And relax, just forget all about it,' was Sally's advice.

'I'm not thinking about it, are you?' I said as we huddled on the beach at Terrigal under the umbrella. 'I'm just not thinking about it. By the way, did you pack the thermometer or did I?'

'Try some different positions,' said my sister. 'That'll get those eggs of yours moving. A bit of the novel and exotic, that's what you need.'

Rubbish. A bit of the novel and exotic just got me moving to the chiropractor.

Some people were also unbelievably insensitive.

'I hate to tell you this, Penny,' said a work colleague with one of those vexing sanctimonious smiles, 'WE got pregnant first time.'

'Oh, WE must be thrilled,' I replied, resisting the urge to head butt her bulging abdomen.

And I'll never forget the moment of revelation when a friend said, 'Oh God, a guy just has to look at me and I get pregnant.'

I raced home. 'Wake up, wake up. Yes, yes, I know you're tired but you don't have to do anything. Just look at me, go on, just look at me!'

But all this well-meant advice proved to be fruitless.

The number of times women boasted about their fertility was extraordinary. They wore it like a badge of honour as if it was somehow the result of hours and hours of study, something they'd worked hard to achieve, rather than a biological quirk that selects its victims at random.

For the non-, sub-, in-, call us what you will, fertile are just that: biological victims. However, it's hard to reconcile nature's quirky little ways with the very real and profound desire to have a child. You can't help but feel that it's your fault. How could something ostensibly as natural as breathing just not function correctly?

'It's not fair,' I would weep. 'ANYONE can have a baby. Why can't I? And why does my period always start the minute after I've done a pregnancy test?'

And so we returned again to the specialist.

'There seem to be no physiological reasons as to why you're not conceiving. Blood tests,' he added cursorily.

'And they will show what exactly?' convinced by now that he thought we were the sort of people who should never have children.

'Blood tests will determine the hormone levels in your body. You may not be producing enough oestrogen to trigger ovulation.'

By now I was really concerned. I'd always believed that I would have a child and yet now I had to start thinking seriously about a childless future. I felt angry and depressed. One minute we'd dream up exotic travel plans, always travelling first class with all the money we'd save by being childless, and the next minute I'd be in tears having to cross the road because I'd spotted a pregnant cat.

When people gave us the nudge, the wink and the

predictable, 'Isn't it time you guys were starting your family,' we'd just say, 'You can't be serious. We hate kids.'

As my periods came and went with monotonous irregularity it took another six months to discover that it was indeed my hormonal system that was proving so uncooperative. The solution to the hormonal imbalance was a fertility drug that has the unfortunate side-effect of an increase in the possibility of multiple births. Each month the drug dose was doubled and we eventually decided that childlessness was preferable to septuplets.

Both low- and high-tech medicine had proven spectacularly unsuccessful in my case and we didn't quite know what to do next. Just before we applied for an overdraft to pay for IVF, a work colleague suggested acupuncture. We were both highly sceptical to say the least, but we'd reached a point where we were prepared to try anything.

'There must be something in it,' said my sister. 'China's the most overpopulated country in the world.'

'They've just got lousy TV,' said my husband.

'I may as well give it a go,' I said. 'After all, one prick is much like another.'

It was a great relief to lie on my back for half an hour and for once not have to do anything interactive, though I couldn't see how hair-fine needles in my shins and wrists were going to convince my ovaries to get their act together.

'I think I might do a pregnancy test tomorrow,' I said after several sessions and no period.

'Don't waste the money. Anyway, it'll only upset us,' said my husband.

I'll never forget standing in the kitchen bellowing up the stairs, 'Come and look at this. I can't believe it. I think I'm pregnant!'

And I was.

The curious thing is that neither of us went into raptures, neither of us was flooded with a joyous ecstasy of overpowering emotion—the sort of thing that always happens to people in movies. We were more stunned than overjoyed. For even though we'd been trying for so long, we had never fully believed that it wouldn't happen, that it *couldn't* happen, so that when it finally did, it was almost something of an anti-climax. I think too that I'd become so determined just to get pregnant, to prove that I could (though who was I trying to impress? the butcher?), that we hadn't actually given much thought to the implications of parenting, to the lifestyle changes that a child inevitably brings.

But the beauty of pregnancy is that you have a long time to get used to the idea, and we did. Fortunately, I had no morning sickness but to compensate had what's called pregnancy rhinitis, which is an inability to breathe because your nasal passages are swollen like the Nile at flood time. It's hideous. Commercial nasal sprays carried warnings about use during pregnancy and I spent vast amounts of time ringing drug companies to find out why. On balance I decided that oxygen deprivation and high stress levels would be far more harmful to my foetus than a little blood vessel constriction.

Like all first-time parents we assiduously attended the antenatal classes and watched the graphic videos, though now I'm of the firm belief that the birth is the least of your worries.

Having been in no hurry to be conceived, our son was similarly in no hurry to be born and he was induced nearly two weeks after his due date. After the prostaglandin gel had been inserted and nothing happened (I was used to that), I ate a piece of chocolate cake and a chicken sandwich and smugly announced to my sister and my husband that I couldn't see what all the fuss was about. After I threw up into the wastepaper basket I then spent the next few hours becoming all too familiar with what all the fuss was about.

I found full-on labour to be an unrelieved and relentlessly painful experience of unspeakable proportions. I vaguely recall my sister urging me to do some pelvic rocking and my husband keeping himself busy tracking down ice packs or hot packs, all of which were singularly useless. I'd liked the idea of a drug-free birth but it remained just that— an idea, a poor idea. The gas was totally ineffectual and I'm convinced that the pethidine might have had some effect had the midwives been a little less stingy with the dose. The epidural was bliss, comparatively speaking, you understand. I have as yet to meet anyone who thoroughly enjoyed their first child's birth.

I was fortunate that my son was induced on 31 March because there can be no greater incentive to push than seeing the clock tick steadily towards midnight and April Fools' Day. He made it with an hour to spare.

It is said that pleasure is the absence of pain, and as that bloodied and mucusy body was eased from mine the relief was exquisite. But he was exquisite too. He was nine pounds, four ounces, boofy just like his father, spotty and prone to cry at the drop of a hat, just like his mother, and we thought he was just extraordinary. And still do.

(A shorter version of this story was first published in the *Australian* 30 May 1995.)

DEBBIE SPILLANE
One Rung Below an Axe-Murderer

I don't think I ever really wanted to be a mother. Since accepting the challenge of putting my thoughts and experiences about motherhood into words, I've wrestled with the implications of coming right out and making that statement. I'm aware how brutal and insensitive it sounds. I feel envious and vaguely isolated when I see and hear how vital, rewarding and inspiring other women find motherhood. I feel guilty because despite a substantial lack of maternal instinct, I've produced two beautiful, intelligent daughters who have to cope with a mother who has never come close to fitting the image that society portrays of what a 'Mum' should be, do and feel.

The circumstances leading up to the birth in 1981 of my first child, Jemima, look quite reasonable, on paper.

At 26 years of age I was a not-too-young and not-too-old mother. I was married, albeit only a few months, when I fell pregnant and it was, as they say, a 'planned pregnancy'. I don't know whether it's a question regularly asked of all pregnant women, or whether my obvious state of shell-shock prompted the enquiry, but I seem to recall everyone asking in confidential tones, 'Was it a planned pregnancy?'

It was, I couldn't deny it. But I hadn't planned it very thoroughly, and certainly hadn't planned on it happening so quickly. All I can say about the whole business is, 'it seemed like a good idea at the time'.

Roger and I had married in 1980 after a relationship of just a few months. I had already been married once, rushing into matrimony at a very unripe 19 years of age. One of the issues that had driven that marriage to an early demise was my lack of interest in having a family. I had a job in the public service, I was studying part-time at university, I was singing in a band and I felt I had any number of interests in life I wanted to pursue ahead of motherhood. I was 21 when that marriage folded.

At 25 I felt like I had my priorities sorted out. My musical interests had overtaken my university studies. I had let my arts degree at Sydney University fizzle out just one subject short of the target. I had taken a job in a record store and was singing in bands. Roger was a record company sales representative who called on the shop I worked in. He was also the guitarist in a band that I ended up joining. We moved in together, we married, we worked during the day and spent our evenings and weekends rehearsing, songwriting and working in pubs and clubs. He was keen to have a family, and I had somehow developed this notion that I could handle motherhood plus all that without any problems. Almost as soon as the idea crossed my mind, bingo! I was pregnant.

At the time I seemed to have met or heard about dozens of couples who were 'trying to start a family' without any luck. The culprit, so popular theory had it, was the contraceptive pill.

'If you've been taking the pill for several years it can take 12 to 18 months after stopping before your cycle returns to normal,' female friends told me. Blithely, I tossed away the little foil packet thinking that maybe I'd get pregnant sometime next year. It turned out to be the very next month.

So it was planned and yet unexpected.

Looking back over my childhood, teens and early 20s I can't remember a time when I ever pictured myself as a mother. I resisted early training, rejecting dolls outright as a little girl. I could never understand how you could've preferred one of them to a teddy bear or pet cat. I was amazed by the fuss other females made about babies. I regarded them as quaint, unattractive little beings with a range of unappealing odours and anti-social habits.

Sure, I thought my youngest brother and sister were cute babies—I was old enough to remember my mother

135

giving birth to both of them, and to be able to help out by giving them bottles and changing nappies occasionally—but as for giving second glances to babies of relatives, or neighbours, or stray ones in strollers at supermarkets . . . no way! Throughout high school I was too busy dreaming of being a jockey, test cricket umpire or football coach to picture a baby on the horizon, and then when I got to university my rock singer ambitions kicked in and, as I didn't see too many bassinets on *Countdown*, motherhood didn't seem relevant. When I heard myself telling friends and family that I was having a baby, I almost felt I was listening to someone else talking.

Cautiously, I admitted to a few close friends that I was a little underwhelmed by the rather sudden onset of motherhood. 'Don't worry,' they counselled. 'Once you get over morning sickness you'll feel more enthused.'

In accordance with the pregnancy handbooks, my morning sickness stopped magically at 12 weeks. I waited for maternal instinct to rear its kindly head. It didn't. Just a sense of unreality colliding with a mixture of adventure and apprehension. 'When you can actually feel the baby moving inside you it'll be different,' they reassured me.

Eventually I started feeling the little elbows and knees prodding, and while this was indeed fascinating, it still wasn't exactly bringing on a warm glow of contentment. I guess it felt more like I was conducting some sort of lab experiment on my own body. I was constantly astonished by the process, and absorbed in reading whatever I could about pregnancy and childbirth, but still basically shocked that it was happening to me.

Something I simply couldn't bring myself to do was attend antenatal classes. No way in the world. It just didn't feel like something I wanted to participate in as a group activity. Like organised worship, or organised workouts, it wasn't for me. In addition to the philosophical objection, there was also the underlying dread of 'the birth video'. To this day I have never watched a video of anyone giving birth and have no desire to. I'm a sook. I used to shut my eyes during episodes of M*A*S*H so I knew a full action preview would definitely panic me. I squirmed enough looking at the still photographs in books. I figured my best chance of staying reasonably calm during labour was to have an intellectual understanding of what was going on without an actual mental picture of the nitty-gritty. I talked to as many mothers as I could about their birth experiences and formed the firm opinion that there was no point having a firm opinion on how I wanted to give birth. I liked the theory of 'natural childbirth' but decided I wasn't making any promises to myself or anyone else about drug-free labour.

Just as well, as it turned out.

Maternal feelings still hadn't overtaken me but by the time I reached the last six weeks of pregnancy I was keen to get the whole motherhood show on the road. Our band, Bluey, had worked in pubs and clubs up until then, with me decked out in large navy King Gee overalls, the closest approximation to cool maternity wear I could find. We hadn't taken bookings inside the last six weeks, though, for fear of having to make a late cancellation. My mother had delivered at least four weeks early with all four of us and I was convinced this was likely in my case. Besides, much as I hated to admit it, I had to slow down. Managing a record store, I was on my feet all day, and then when the band worked at night, I was hoofing it till midnight or later and the pace was starting to tell. I was slumping in a chair between sets, legs cramping and aching.

I will never forget an incident at a western suburbs pub—during a break, as the DJ pumped out recorded music, a punter asked me if I wanted to dance. 'Sorry, but I'm really tired,' I explained, apologetically. 'Aw c'mon! Get into it a bit!' he remonstrated with me. 'Seriously, I can't. I'm seven months pregnant,' I replied with exasperation. 'Are ya? Geez, thought you was pullin' a bit of extra weight!' he declared and wandered off, stubby in hand, shaking his head.

But once the band stopped working, and I quit the shop—a sad move for me because I'd only just progressed to being manager—I was crawling the walls. The only activity that stopped me from going completely stir crazy was band practice. We had decided to use the opportunity to rehearse some new material and it was a rehearsal that kept me up till midnight the day before I went into labour, a labour that didn't resemble any of the models my research had turned up.

I woke around four am with what felt like mild period pain. I had gone two days past my due date and was alert to any twinge or twitch. As I'd done a few times in previous days, I looked at the clock and made a note of the time in case the pain reappeared. It did, after about three minutes. Again three minutes after that. And again after about the same interval. According to my reading, if the pains were three minutes apart I needed to get to the hospital, but as it was more like discomfort than real pain I knew that would be overreacting. Even though we had the Scrabble board on stand-by and the hospital bag packed, I was determined not to spend unnecessary hours hanging around a hospital. I decided to ignore it and try to build on my four hours' sleep in case the action heated up. Nice idea, but the combination of nervous excitement and a decent sort of pain in the belly every three minutes made sleep impossible.

I decided to get up, have a shower then call the hospital for advice. Trouble was, when I got up and starting walking around, the pain eased considerably. It was still there, every three minutes or so, but it was hardly worth mentioning. Whenever I lay down, it hurt more. So by 5.30 am I was up for the day. By six that night I was thinking it was all some sort of sick joke. The three minute routine had kept up all day. I'd tried lying down several times only to be forced back up by immediate intensification of the pain. I'd been shopping late in the day, leaning on the trolley every few minutes as the pain gradually got stronger.

Everyone I talked to said, 'Must be false labour. With the real thing when the pains get to three minutes apart you won't have any doubt what's going on.'

After dinner that night I finally rang the hospital. Although I wasn't convinced this was it, I knew I couldn't sleep and wanted to know what to do. 'You'd better come in,' they said, warning in the same breath that it was possibly false labour. I didn't hurry, but using the bathroom shortly before leaving home I noticed a show of blood. 'Great,' I thought. 'If this is the real thing maybe the pains will start spacing out to about 30 or at least 20 minutes apart.'

No such luck.

At nine pm I arrived at the hospital. A brusque midwife told me I had 'hours and hours to go yet', and should get some sleep. But with what now felt like extreme period pain every three minutes, that seemed a ridiculous suggestion. Roger and I played Scrabble in the waiting room (he beat me too, the heartless bastard!) but after a couple of hours I was exhausted.

'Take these sleeping pills,' the midwife advised.

'Will I actually be able to sleep?' I asked suspiciously, looking at the unwelcoming steel-frame bed and linoleum floor.

'Sure. You'll need to. You've got a long day ahead of you.' That sort of dire prediction after 19 hours of contractions three minutes apart, made me want to cry. About half an hour after taking the sleeping pills I *was* crying. I was a zombie. Nodding off and then being woken again every three minutes was like some form of torture. The contractions were lasting longer and whatever energy I'd had left to fight the pain had been sapped by the sleeping pills. I was a sobbing mess.

I tried the gas but all that did was make me feel so stoned and vague I kept forgetting what the hell was going on. I'd have a painful contraction and think, 'Shit! What's that? Oh that's right, I'm having a baby!'

By four am I was just whimpering constantly and pitifully about wanting sleep. Someone told me the only way to ensure that was to have an epidural. The prospect of having an injection in the spine had always seemed totally unthinkable, but at this point if someone had suggested I could sleep after being hit on the head with a lump of four-by-two, I would've agreed.

The injection hurt, but I remember thinking how nice it was to feel a different pain. After that the sensation was quite remarkable. I felt like I was being filled up with iced water from the waist down. Gradually the pain disappeared and I drifted off. When I woke only a couple of hours later I felt fresh, relieved and excited about the impending birth of our baby. Before the epidural a midwife had warned me it might delay the birth. She was saying I was maybe still eight or more hours away from being fully dilated. When I woke I complained of feeling pressure on my vagina. The midwife checked me out and said, 'Oh, it's the baby's head.'

The same thing happened nine years later when I was giving birth to Eleanor. I asked (nay, pleaded!) for an epidural, and was warned it might slow the labour. Within an hour I was rested and ready to move into the final stage. Politically incorrect it might be, but I'm an epidural fan. Another midwife confided later on that they are bound to give warnings about delaying effects with epidurals although it's reasonably common for the painkiller to relax the mother so much that labour speeds up.

Anyway, back to the birth of Jemima. After a few hours of huffing, puffing, pushing and panting, I started to get a bit wheezy. Being an asthmatic, I asked Roger to find my Ventolin inhaler. This seemed to throw the medical staff into panic. 'She's getting asthmatic,' someone gasped. 'Better get the doctor.' Within minutes an obstetrician appeared, suggested a low forceps delivery and asked whether a throng of students (I was a public outpatient at a teaching hospital) could watch the final minutes of play.

I couldn't have cared less. As long as it meant it was going to be over shortly, I would've agreed to being wheeled out, feet in stirrups, into the centre of the MCG with every grandstand full, a giant replay screen, the works. I just wanted it over. And very quickly it was. By 11 am I had a beautiful baby girl with a thick mop of black hair that, after washing, turned out to be streaked with ginger. The streaks didn't last long, unfortunately, but she still has amazingly thick, dark brown hair. These days she dyes it black.

One of my most enduring memories of that morning was hearing my mother's voice in the corridor outside the delivery room. She was quite panicky because I'd been in labour so long, and was anxiously demanding to know what was going on. She was my first visitor after Jemima's birth and my greatest asset in the months that followed.

Having encouraged me to go back and finish my last arts subject at uni, she volunteered to babysit the few hours a week I needed to attend classes. With mid-year assignments and 'take-home' exams (definitely *not* designed for new mothers) due only six weeks or so after Jemima's birth, I thought I would have a breakdown. I wanted to drop out, again. Mum came over one day and gave me a lecture about not giving up my life for my children. 'Even if you give up everything for them, they'll never really appreciate it, and you'll end up bitter,' she declared.

I sometimes wonder if I took her advice further than she meant me to.

Two-and-a-half years later, Roger and I split up, and, after a few months of trying it the more socially acceptable way, we decided Jemima should live with him. I had started work as a sports journalist with unpredictable hours. In any case, even before that, I had long since given over primary carer duties to him. I craved a career. He'd been supporting himself since he was 16 and was far more interested in family and fatherhood than the vagaries of the record business.

Jemima was seven years old and wearing a black-checked dress when she played flower girl at the registry office wedding between Greg and me in 1988. We had met working at 2DAY-FM in Sydney. He was an announcer, I was sports reporter on the breakfast show.

This time, I thought, I'll get my motherhood act together. Greg already had a son, Christopher, from a previous relationship but was basically being denied access (illegally) by a difficult mother. I suppose, looking back on it, subconsciously we were both in a hurry to prove ourselves good parents.

I can't believe I managed to shock myself the same way twice. Within a few months of getting married we decided to have a baby. When I stopped taking the pill I had one period, then I was pregnant.

It turned out to be poor timing. The radio station was bought out by a bigger company. There were predictions of radical staff changes. I was petrified. A pregnant sports reporter seemed a soft target. I kept it secret for as long as I could, although surreptitiously combining morning sickness with 5.30 am starts wasn't easy. Eventually the truth, like my waistline, had to come out.

'Not a problem,' the management dude told me. 'They like you.'

I had nine weeks of holidays owing and agreed to take them from Christmas through till mid-February. The baby was due mid-January. I would be back at work a week after the first survey of 1990—an all important consideration in radio terms. Everyone seemed happy with the arrangement—it made nice publicity for the station, after all.

My pregnancy, like the one nearly 10 years before, was uneventful. Morning sickness stopped like clockwork at 12 weeks, I enjoyed keeping busy, and a desk job was much easier on the body than the shop and band duties I'd survived first time around. But emotionally it got a bit rocky near the end.

A week before I left for my 'holidays', two of the other three members of the breakfast team were sacked. I was curious, unsettled, nervous about what shape my job would take the next year, but meantime I had Christmas and a baby to prepare for so I had enough distractions. Oddly enough the action all started in the kitchen at the radio station.

I was two days overdue and worried about being home on my own when Greg was on-air. 2DAY-FM was only five minutes from my hospital so we'd decided it might be simpler if I spent the four hours this particular Sunday watching cricket in the newsroom while Greg worked. Early in the afternoon I went to the kitchen to make a cup of tea and, while chatting with one of the newsroom guys, felt a sudden gush of warm water down the inside of my leg. People joke that I can talk through anything, and I did. I figured if I didn't react he wouldn't notice. He didn't, but as soon as possible I shored up the damage and rushed into the studio to tell Greg. We waited for labour pains to begin. Nothing.

He finished his shift, we came home, nothing. I rang the hospital, and they told me to come straight in. I wasn't keen. I knew how long it had taken last time, even after the pains had started. I made a pact with myself that I'd go to the hospital after Mark Taylor reached his century in the Test that was being televised. He did. Still no labour pains. I switched over to the men's final of the NSW Open tennis. That finished and still no labour pains. I rang the hospital again and they got quite stroppy about the fact that I hadn't already presented myself for inspection. They started talking infections. Reluctantly we toddled off.

After an examination we settled in to watch more TV in the hospital waiting room. By 10 pm they were suggesting I get a good night's sleep and look forward to an induction in the morning. Sweet dreams!

At around 11 pm the pains started. Three minutes apart.

'Here we go again,' I thought.

Sure enough they stayed that way throughout the night. They had started with more oomph than in my first labour and by four am I was starting to struggle. I asked for an epidural. 'Your wife's doing fine,' they told my husband when around five am he relayed the message that I wanted an epidural. 'Says WHO?' I seem to remember howling. 'I am NOT fucking fine!'

Around six am they relented and gave me an epidural. I dozed a little then woke only an hour later with a burning pain. The baby had travelled down the birth canal, and suddenly it was action stations. The epidural seemed to have been administered more sparingly this time around. They told me it was designed to wear out during delivery and it sure did. This birth was more painful, but quicker and didn't require forceps. Eleanor was born at around 8.30 am and, as with Jemima's birth, my mum was hovering in the corridor in time to be my first visitor.

I enjoyed the early weeks of motherhood much more on the second occasion. Eleanor started sleeping through the night within days of coming home and I felt none of the stress and pressure I'd encountered with Jemima. I can remember just sitting around holding her while she slept, feeling at ease and more contented with the role of mother.

That changed within about a fortnight.

My father-in-law phoned one Sunday morning and asked if I had read the radio column in the Sunday paper. I hadn't. He wouldn't say what it was about but a quick trip to the newsagent soon revealed all. The radio station had announced that the guy filling in for me had been given my job permanently. The general manager was quoted saying he thought a part-time job would be more suitable for me anyway now that I had a baby. He said options would be discussed with me when I was 'well enough'.

I had been 'well enough' up until then. I wasn't for a while after that. The decision, and the way I found out about it, threw me into a fit of depression. To make matters worse there were also question marks over Greg's job. He'd been demoted to midnight-to-dawn, just perfect for a new dad. Suddenly our contentment had turned to insecurity and bitterness.

I returned to my new part-time job after my nine weeks' 'holiday' but was retrenched two months later. Six months later Greg was sacked. Not long afterwards I started working on *Live & Sweaty* as well as on a Newcastle radio station, while Greg worked part-time. It was just the way the cards fell at the time. It meant again I had handed over the role of primary carer to my husband.

When we separated six years later it seemed crazy to split Greg and Eleanor up. Besides, once again, I was working the offbeat hours. Doing *Hard Coffee* on Triple J, I wasn't getting home until eight each night and, as a sports columnist, my weekends were full-on sport.

My mum always used to say that my girls were the only toddlers she ever knew who used to cry, 'I want my daddy!' if they fell over or got upset. That amused me, as well as hurt a little. I've tried to figure it out many times. When a mother elects to leave a child with its father there's a constant need to justify it—to yourself and the rest of society. To have done it twice seems generally to put you about one rung below an axe-murderer on the social acceptability ladder.

My only defence is to say that, with all honesty, I never really saw myself as a mother. I often wonder if I should not have had children, but in the same breath I have to say I could never regret it. I'm proud of my daughters and extremely grateful to their excellent fathers. I see heaps of both Jemima and Eleanor but I am painfully aware of how much of a mum I am not.

Nothing could have brought that home to me more than the death of my own mother last year. A wise, warm, generous and hard-working woman, she somehow managed to raise and help support four of us. She went on to build a career starting in her mid-40s, only to die at 60 when she was looking forward to retirement.

I remember when the four of us stood around her body, having listened to and watched those final breaths, each taking a turn at saying goodbye. I hadn't thought about what to say but I found myself whispering, 'Thanks Mum, you did a fantastic job.'

Maybe each of us take for granted the things that come too easily to us. I know my mum would've liked me to be a better mother. All I can say is I guess there were lots of other things I learned from her. I hope one day my girls will feel the same about me.

FIONA GILES
Two Breasts, Twelve Weeks

First Days

This is something I know I can do. Yet when I express my first drops of colostrum, propped up in bed at Beth Israel Hospital, I am amazed at this proof that my breasts actually work. After shamelessly admiring them since I was 14, I am delighted to confirm that they have not just been perched there for my narcissistic indulgence, nor merely as the Scylla and Charybdis of hopeful men.

The lactation consultant has called by at my request, her big-sisterly demeanour a welcome contrast to the scratchy collection of nurses and medical technicians. Her encouraging voice flows soothingly through my drugged brain as she arranges her fingers around my nipple and rolls them across my areola so that creamy fluid drips into a tiny medication cup. Having a strange woman's hands on me should be odd but it isn't, since I am looking at my breasts as entirely new things. They could almost be someone else's. They are much larger than mine. They are mapped by inky veins suggesting a well-endowed river basin. And if I cross my arms I have a cleavage. I am fully qualified to just say no to the Wonderbra rack at Macy's.

The lactation consultant now demonstrates a let-down massage, her fingers spiralling around my breast in a series of tiny circles, then tracing feathery lines inward in a clockwise direction. Richard walks in and, exuberant with my achievement, I dip my finger in the cup to taste my early milk, which is as warm as melted butter. Holding out my finger, I ask Richard if he would like to try some. He takes two steps back and pulls a face, as if I'd offered him a dead frog. I guess it's a bit early to explore the erotic potential of my new toys.

Brodie is downstairs in the Neo-natal Intensive Care Unit, where he will stay for the next three days. Delivered by emergency C-section at 35 weeks, he needs extra oxygen, an IV drip and constant monitoring. Four days earlier I had been doing leg lifts at Maternal Fitness class when I haemorrhaged, making an impressive mess in the white gymnasium. I caught a taxi straight to the hospital where placenta praevia was diagnosed. A tiny part of the placenta was covering my cervix, effectively blocking the baby's exit. The sonogram also showed that the baby was a footling breech. One of these conditions was enough to make surgery inevitable. So much for a trillion Kegels.

An eleventh-hour amniocentesis to check for foetal lung maturity indicated the need to delay delivery for another week, and after two days in hospital I was sent home and ordered to stay in bed. But within 24 hours I was bleeding again. So here I was with waistline restored, staples for a bikini line and, somewhere nearby, a baby.

I should by now be beside myself with longing for Brodie, if I weren't already beside myself in a morphine haze, woozily regarding this new, deranged mother-person. That the nurses keep addressing me as mommy, as in 'How's mommy doing?', doesn't help to make me feel more myself.

The piece of me that still inhabits my body is obsessed by the need to establish breastfeeding. This piece sticks firm to the hope of salvaging a remnant of my earth-crunchy fantasy from the hospital's high-tech coup. I am grateful to the staff and their technology for delivering Brodie safely, but I feel a sense of loss from undergoing surgery and from being separated from my child. Hence my first sign of real joy at this evidence of my body performing as expected.

While Brodie and I are each detained in our separate quarters by electronic monitors and IV drips, Richard is bonding by proxy. I have a Polaroid taken by the intensive care staff. My spirits depend on Richard spending as much time as possible reassuring Brodie that life holds more than harsh lights, needles and high-pitched beeps. Meanwhile, I practise with the hospital's Medela electric pump, expressing small amounts from each breast for the intensive care nurses to feed him during the night. I feel ridiculous but defiant making these tiny offerings and none of the nurses thinks to assure me that a teaspoon of colostrum is nutritionally superior to an ounce of formula, a fact I've forgotten in my embarrassment.

Twenty-four hours after surgery, when I'm allowed to sit up and can walk a few steps, I ask Richard to take me in a wheelchair to the intensive care nursery so we can begin feeding. By now we are adept at dodging my plastic tubing and manoeuvring the chair, but as Richard bends down to secure the foot pedals, one of them breaks off in his hand, exposing a jagged metal edge. Stupidly, I forget to be indignant that this expensive private teaching hospital should be so run down, and wonder where we can hide the broken part. Having already encountered cockroaches in the wash-basin, broken blinds, and other hallmarks of shoddy motels, I shouldn't be surprised by this new development.

Downstairs is little better. No space is set aside for breastfeeding in the crowded so-called nursery, so we deposit ourselves in a tiny adjacent office which seems to function as a dumping ground for disused furniture and equipment. Crammed between a water cooler and a rubbish bin, I hold out my arms for the silent bundle, who exhibits a Zen-like imperviousness to his surroundings.

I had seen Brodie only briefly before being taken to my room after surgery: once when he was flashed past my eyes in the operating room; the second time when I'd insisted on my right to be wheeled into the intensive care unit on my way upstairs. Already throwing up from the morphine, I started to cry on seeing him lying there so calm and alone, all wired up. When I had then reached out to touch him I had been asked not to as my hand was inadvertently interfering with the pathway of an electronic sensor.

So now is our chance finally to touch. Having been together for nine months, the sudden separation of the past day has been a rude shock, and our reunion is dramatically comforting. My pain lifts miraculously and Brodie's breathing becomes stronger.

My immediate challenge is to arrange myself and Brodie around the various wires and tubing. For the first few moments I fumble like an abandoned puppet, striving to support Brodie's head and to position him securely while avoiding the incision in my stomach. In past months I have studied so many illustrations of breastfeeding holds—the 'football hold' (recommended for caesar mothers), the clutch, the cradle, lying down, doing it while pushing your shopping trolley through the canned food aisle—that I was sure this would be a snap. Instead, I am made timid by fear of dropping him or of dislodging the cumbersome wooden splint that secures the drip in his arm.

Worse than anything, my breast seems bigger than his head. Brodie's mouth cannot possibly take hold of my mountainous nipple, let alone get a proper mouthful of breast, which must loom over him like a ghostly zeppelin. In contrast to my panic, he maintains his meditative poise and makes barely a sound. Eyes scrunched tight against the lights, he valiantly searches for my nipple, and I tickle his cheek to help him find it. Stuffing my breast into his mouth, in the one or two seconds at a time that he opens wide, is harder than it appeared in the books. His head is not only tiny, but wobbly, and I'm not used to deploying my breast as a battering ram. He succeeds in latching on once or twice, and sucks briefly, but is soon overcome by tiredness. Discouraged by my uselessness, and fearful that the nurses pushing formula have corrupted his urge to suckle, I decide that we should just sleep and cuddle.

It is here that my mother finds us later that day, having booked a flight from Perth to New York as soon as she heard I was in hospital. I point out our problem. I am the monster mother, Mrs Bates, the north face my son has to scale.

Taking my breast in one hand and Brodie's head in the other, she quietly plants us together.

Week One
This is where humans learn how to kiss. The happy confusion of food and love brings orality's ultimate gift.

The mother's nipple is the baby's first toy, and breastfeeding his first challenge. Later my baby will find his thumb, then toys and solid food. Later still, he will discover a cigarette or, if he's luckier, a cerebral substitute. (If he becomes a father, he might celebrate the moment by sucking on a cigar.)

But most of all, he will seek to encounter a warm face and re-enact the old game, pausing to grapple with someone who returns the same blind wishes.

He will again become speechless.

Week Two
8 pm RB (8.30); 11 pm LB (11.30); 1 am RB (1.15); 3 am LB (?); 5.30 am RB (10 min); (LB 7.30?); 8 am RB; 10.30 am LB; 1 pm RB; 3 pm LB; 5.45 pm RB (LB & RB); 8.15 pm LB; 11 pm RB; 12.30 am LB; 4 am RB & LB; 6.30 am?; 8.30 am RB & LB; 11 am LB & RB; 2.15 pm Grandma 60 ml; 4.45 pm RB (6.30); 7.30 pm RB; 10.15 pm LB ...

Richard and Mum insist I have a break at night by allowing them to take over one feed. We agree on using supplemental finger feeding so that Brodie doesn't succumb to nipple confusion or begin to prefer the more passive action used for feeding from a bottle. The system uses a nipple which extends into a fine plastic tube taped to the little finger, so that Brodie is fed like a poddy calf. It is designed for mothers who produce only a little milk or who have adopted a baby but want to mimic breastfeeding. The bottle is therefore designed to hang around the mother's neck with the tubing taped to her nipple.

Enlisting gravity to aid the flow of milk, Richard clips his bottle to the peak of his baseball cap. Mum clips hers to the curtain. I get the impression they could do this all day and night if only I would let them.

The exhilaration of bringing Brodie home is beginning to wane, and at the start of each evening I dread the interruptions to come. But it turns out that each night is not long and tedious at all and bears none of the anxiety or boredom of insomnia. Instead, it is a series of drifting chapters, and, as we slip in and out of sleeping and feeding, the two states are barely distinguishable. Oxytocin, the hormone that stimulates milk production, has an added tranquillizing effect. I float in and out of sleep in the rocking chair as Brodie sucks, then wake to take him into bed until morning. The paediatrician has instructed me to ensure he's fed at least once every three hours. I note down the times, but even so, by daylight, it's difficult to recall any details.

For the first time in my life since I was myself a child, I am living entirely in the present. It is a huge relief.

Week Three
Mum has left. She cooked dinner for us every night for two weeks. I can't imagine life without her.

Brodie gags on my breastmilk and I'm sure he will choke and die. How can I explain this to his paediatrician? I wonder if there are any documented cases of mothers drowning their babies with sudden let-down. But who would own up to it?

Eyes bugging and gasping for air, he rallies and comes back for a second try. I take this as conclusive evidence that my son is a survivor.

Every time Brodie latches on still feels like a small miracle of energy, instinct and determination. I am sometimes producing too much milk between feeds and have to pump for a minute or two to soften my breasts, so that he can get a grip more easily. He sucks furiously to stimulate the milk ejection reflex, then slows down to swallow as the milk comes in. He works hard, and sometimes breaks out in a sweat from the effort. All his energy is focused on clenching his jaw and working his tongue to draw my nipple up against his palate. He rests frequently, which at first worried me, but now I know it's just his style. After each pause, his chin begins to tremble as he musters his forces.

This week I discovered I can walk around while breastfeeding, to answer the phone or retrieve a glass of water. I can also breastfeed and eat dinner while talking on the phone. I feel fabulously proud of these feats. Even so, I prefer to do nothing but sit on the sofa and gaze upon him while he feeds.

Our relationship is centred around perfecting our skills. It's virtually all we do.

Week Four

I've been explaining to Brodie that you can't be too thin or too rich, as he's still on the slender side and would look chic in tight black jeans. Nevertheless, I am hoping the paediatrician will congratulate me on his weight gain. In New York there are no community-based child health centres, where I might check his weight or ask the advice of a matronly nurse, or just hang out with other mothers. Instead, I must wait for each, now monthly, visit to the paediatrician, saving my list of questions for the big day.

After a normal, but still disappointing loss of more ounces since leaving hospital, he has at last turned around, and is now nearly eight pounds. His thinness emphasises the importance of my role as provider, so that all my energy is galvanised to this single physical task. I am also fuelled by guilt at having caused him to be yanked into the world before he'd had a chance to store some fat of his own.

Breastfeeding is the most elemental of relationships and a baby's first social act, ensuring the ultimate success of the reproductive drama. My competence depends on nothing but my accessibility and my milk supply, and my baby's ability to stimulate that supply by sucking. With the advent of formula it is no longer strictly true that humans depend on breastfeeding for survival. But when it works, breastfeeding mounts a relationship between bodies based purely on physical interaction. Its psychosomatic give-and-take makes it a form of congress not unlike procreative sex.

Freud writes, 'Sucking at his mother's breast has become the prototype of every relation of love.' The relationship with my son, growing out of these days and nights, will in large part be shaped by this dance, just as intercourse between lovers is an extension of, a departure from, and a forging ground for their interaction as a whole.

It is well known that lactation slides against eros, and the breast goes on to become central to adult sexuality, which is one reason public breastfeeding can be controversial. (Another reason is the taboo against performing a bodily function in public, except for eating. It's OK to see things going into our bodies but not to see anything coming out. Even tears can cause social consternation.) There are both hormonal and neurological connections between the nipples, the uterus and the clitoris. At the evolutionary level this is logical, since, if breastfeeding wasn't pleasurable, what mother would be persuaded by her baby's cries to feed 12 or more times a day, despite exhaustion, pain and the needs of other children? At the physiological level, the breast protects the heart; and used as a singular noun, it is the facade for the vital organs. Both metaphorically and literally, the breast of either sex promises love and comfort. And its ambient beat keeps constant, bittersweet time, a reminder of mortality.

Yet breastfeeding also exists securely in its own maternal orbit. This place is more cannibalistic than erotic. As the baby eats, it leeches nourishment from one body to another—so startlingly effective a procedure, it seems feasible to sit and watch a baby grow. This economy between mother and child is atavistic enough to render the sexual journey of sperm to ova relatively abstract.

Having read about women who have orgasms while feeding their babies, I am on the lookout for my own sexual response. But I don't feel anything more than a quiet sensual pleasure mingled with a sense of grace in being so closely linked to Brodie's needs. It's difficult to describe the sensation caused by the pinching, massaging and pulling of my erectile tissue—except to suppose that it might feel similar to the fellating of a tiny penis. Because I have virtually no oestrogen in my system, my libido is almost non-existent, and I guess that oxytocin on its own isn't sufficient, at this stage, to achieve orgasm. Perhaps mothers who do reach orgasm have already started to wean and to ovulate. Even though I detect no overt sexual response, breastfeeding is still a glorious feeling. Based on a pleasure in abundance, it is without the urgency of climax or closure. The more my baby sucks, the more milk I produce. Conducted in perfect silence, breastfeeding defines plenitude. Its meaning exceeds words as it forever overflows intended ends.

Week Five
Brodie has developed a form of nipple torture, pulling off before he's broken the seal and making a popping sound

as he stretches my nipple to its limit before letting go. At other times he becomes confused by tiredness, not sure if he needs to burp or sleep or feed some more. I am even more clueless, although I can sympathise with his state. Our idyll turns into a tiny battleground and it's hard not to think that he has a particular rage against my breast as he shakes his head while holding on with his mouth, and cries and pushes against me with his clenched fist. Then abruptly, mid-scream, he falls asleep.

I wonder if he's not only confused by tiredness but also feeling his first angst. Having laboured so far to perfect this act, could he be asking himself if this is all there is? Although he returns each time with the renewal of a simple need, perhaps there's also something Sisyphean about the task.

During these frustrating, drawn-out feeds, I plan what I'll do once he's settled, stressed as much by my need to work as by my need to comfort him. But when he finally succumbs to sleep, he is too heavenly to relinquish.

Ambivalence forgotten, he smiles and smiles.

Week Six

Why does all the literature on breastfeeding begin with dire warnings about how difficult breastfeeding can be and how every mother should expect to suffer? Why does my friend tell me how her friend told her that it feels like having your nipples sliced off with a razor blade?

Engorgement ... not enough milk ... too much milk ... thrush ... mastitis ... aching deltoids ... a joyless festival of pain. At the very least I expected having to nurse through the agony of cracked nipples as they adjusted to constant use. Yet at most I feel a mild soreness which goes away within the first minute of each feeding. I have to admit it: my baby has great technique.

Even the famous let-down sensations are mild, just a few seconds of tingling, needle-sharp pains about half a minute after Brodie latches on, or, if I'm away from him, indicating that it's feeding time. It's true that I still leak from one breast when the other is being used, and I get through a T-shirt a night. But I'm promised that this will pass.

I've been wondering about the irresistible thirst I feel when let-down occurs, and my simultaneous loss of appetite. The pinch of Brodie's mouth sends my body a signal to replenish fluids to make more milk, and to stop eating so he can begin. Maybe it is also introjection of his thirst so that I identify more intensely with his needs.

Once Brodie is replete, he falls back against my arm, his head supported in one of my hands. Like a drunk at a picnic, his arms flop sideways and his newly minted double chin sinks down. Amazed by his cool, I have to remind myself that this should not be taken entirely as a sign of trust since Brodie still imagines he is part of me. I suspect my body also entertains this delusion of unity. Although I fear dropping him literally, I have to remember that, as he emerges as a fully cognizant being, he will figuratively drop into that friable package of consciousness called a self.

Week Seven

I push the pram to Toys 'R' Us at Union Square, looking for a crib mirror. As I search haplessly through the tiers of plastic gadgetry, Brodie gets hungry. I find the rest room but there's nowhere to feed him, not even a chair. I plonk myself down on the floor, using the wall to support my back, and give Brodie his snack.

Feeding in public is becoming less stressful. I don't expect to be harassed in Manhattan for something as tame as breastfeeding, given that I'd be competing for attention against genuinely colourful and practised weirdoes. And New York is one of nine states that have passed legislation protecting breastfeeding mothers from harassment. I'm also worrying less about exposing my breasts to the world, to the extent that I could be called shameless. Yet shameless is exactly the case, since there is no reason for embarrassment; and if I look brazen it's because I am completely unapologetic and without regret. As much as parenting is a noble vocation, breastfeeding is a reminder of its narcissistic motives. Not only are my genes worth replicating, I am willing to 'bare my breast' in public to prove my commitment to this cause.

Last week, at a sidewalk café in Gramercy Park, I forgot

to refasten my buttons and bra after feeding, partly because I was engrossed in Brodie and in protecting his head from the sharp-edged tables. But it was also because I find it difficult to do up my bra under my shirt with one hand, balance Brodie in the crook of my other arm, and at the same time not expose more of my body. In all the many books I've read about breastfeeding, none offers advice on how best to manage this part. Only one book has given any tips on dressing, pointing out that a shirt is best unbuttoned from the bottom, so that the top button remains fastened and shields the chest. Stretchy T-shirts and jumpers work best because, pulled up, they still offer cover, and there are no buttons to worry about. My favourite breastfeeding top is a dark green Replay shirt with mother-of-pearl press studs. A shirt with an upside-down zip down the front would be ideal.

Other cultures are less concerned about mothers exposing their breasts and less anxious about breastfeeding's sensual pleasure. In Borneo, mothers see no need to button up after breastfeeding and are implicitly permitted to leave their breasts free of clothing after tending their children and returning to work. Breastfeeding breasts are not considered erotic and are therefore as neutral as an elbow. It is so universal and familiar that a child will simply pull out its mother's breast, or lift up her shirt, when it's hungry. In Bali, a man offered his breast to a baby when there was no mother present. He didn't lactate, but provided a comforting surrogate nipple.

Recently in Connecticut a mother was ordered by a police officer to move on when she had parked in a car park to breastfeed her baby. She drove to police head-quarters to complain and later received an apology from the Police Department, while mothers in the area staged a 'breast-in' at a local deli and a senator introduced a bill guaranteeing Connecticut mothers the right to breastfeed in public. In 1992 a Chicago mother approached a counselling service, concerned about the sexual feelings breastfeeding aroused. Her inquiry led to her being charged with child abuse and neglect, for which she was sent to jail and separated from her child for a year.

Because mothering is so cloistered in the west, breast-feeding is exotic and—to some—disturbing. The idea that an infant might also take sensual pleasure in its mother's body is confusing to an age which has only recently owned up to the prevalence of parent-child incest. Caught in a zealous fervour, we are in danger of making affectionate touch the next taboo.

I find that friends who openly watch Brodie feeding are more relaxing to be with than those who resolutely lock into my gaze or look away.

Week Eight

After hours and hours of holding Brodie I no longer see him as small, but as a squirmy armful, a substantial baby-weight filling my lap. When Richard comes home from work, I hand him over and suddenly he shrinks.

Richard, on the other hand, grows bigger by the day. He walks in the door after work and seems to have grown into a giant. Later, while breastfeeding in the rocking chair, I glance at him lying on the bed watching television and get a shock to see how huge his legs have grown.

As for my own body, I'm still not used to its new silhouette. Since I have burgeoned from 34B to 36DD, I have banished all my stripy T-shirts to the back of the drawer. Although I understand the appeal of large breasts, they don't do it for me. I guess I have too assiduously cultivated a minimalist persona.

I have been proposed to on Spring Street. Otherwise sensible men go hubba hubba. I am a walking picnic.

Week Nine
This week is the deadline for submitting an edited manuscript. I return the pages in time, but not without tiring myself out. Brodie picks up on my stress and frets from one to three am. He seems to need sleep but when I put him in the cot he cries and wants to feed, only to pummel my breast and yell heartbreakingly. I hear the sound of fingernails on a blackboard and realise I'm gritting my teeth. When I finally give up and get Richard to hold him, he falls asleep in seconds. So do I.

Once or twice this week, for the first time since he was

born, I have not been consumed by the novel awareness that I am a mother. I have momentarily 'forgotten' that Brodie exists. When I do remember him it is with a jolt of guilt. Is he OK? Will he disappear or come to harm if I'm not thinking of him? Is my preoccupation with Brodie like an endless *gesundheit*?

I have to remind myself that my thoughts are not a shield and that his life is not dependent on an effort of my imagination.

Week Ten

I am dreamily gazing at the whorl of Brodie's ear and wondering at its preternatural perfection. Using my fingernail, I gently scrape a film of wax from the uppermost furrow, just as I would from my own ear.

As I look for a suggestion of his grown-up features in his baby face, I wonder if I will seek out the ghost of the baby when he's older. When he rages at me as a teenager, will I remember how complete he was when I held him sleeping in my hands?

Through breastfeeding I am learning the meaning of intimacy. It is not so much the tender exchange of confidence or touch, or the intensity of passionate sex, as the simple intimation of need without words.

Brodie and I know each other now better than we ever will.

Week Eleven

Brodie still feeds every two hours and has slept for a maximum of only four hours at one stretch. I wonder if I'm doing something wrong, but decide not to alter my basic strategy of letting him set the pace. He's gaining weight steadily, and is now over 12 pounds. The paediatrician charts his statistics and tells me he has shot up from the fifth percentile at six weeks to the 50th. I ask her if I should try and space his feeds further apart and she says no. What he's doing is what he needs, she says. Breastfeeding represents the pinnacle of our accomplishments.

Seeing how frequently my son needs to feed, I am full of rage at the generation of mothers and their experts who were bullied into feeding their babies only once every four hours. No wonder so many of our generation have eating disorders. We were all raised under the impression that there wasn't enough food to go around.

Evolutionary biologists have theorised that humans are born developmentally underqualified for survival compared to other mammals. This is because humans have such large heads. If we were allowed to grow older in the uterus, there would be no way we could fit through our mother's birth canal. The breast is therefore not just a means to feed, it ensures that we are locked into a nutritional loop, something also suggested by the colostrum and early milk of mothers of premature babies being different in composition from mothers of full-term babies.

The purity of the exchange highlights the ongoing role of the breast in mediating between the mother and her child, and between the child and its world.

The much-vaunted human longing to return to the womb is perhaps not entirely a romantic conceit, since we must carry with us a shadowy grievance concerning our premature eviction. By ensuring access to the mother's body, breastfeeding attempts to make amends for this rude beginning. Scientists hypothesise that another nine months of foetal growth would be ideal. Interestingly, it is between six and nine months that babies begin to experience separation anxiety.

Week Twelve

Brodie has discovered his hands and sucks his fingers, either singly or together, making delicious lip-smacking noises. Sometimes he manages to cram in a thumb as well, or isolates it for advanced thumb-sucking practice.

He was born with one of his hands in his mouth and at first would chew his fist to signal hunger, only exchanging it for my breast. But now he seeks out his hand for fun; and for the first time I can't be sure if he's telling me he's hungry or if he's simply sucking for his own delectation.

He is beginning to realise that he has parts set aside for his exclusive use and that the other parts, which come and go, can be evaluated, measured and stored away.

DONNA MCDONALD
I am a Mother

Once upon a time, when the sun was bright and the sky was blue, I was enchantingly pregnant. I gave birth to a caramel-skinned boy with frowning stern eyes. My newborn son thrived on my love in a home of music and joy.

Then, one day, I woke to discover my only son—just five months old—dead in his cot. My life as a mother had imploded: it was over.

Or so I thought.

This happened a long time ago. Jack would be 10 years old next January. My memory's images of Jack are now blurred. Sometimes I need to breathe his name to myself, to feel the sharpness of its 'ack ack' sound on my lips and tongue, pricking its path to my heart. I imagine myself encased by the steely mesh of my love for my absent son.

The constancy of my need to honour Jack both drives and wearies me: I am unremitting in my efforts to fill the space left behind when he died, a space whose shape teasingly eludes me.

My clarity in recognising this search belies the wrenching difficulty I have in finding the right words, even the right tone, to describe my mother-without-child life. I can talk about my feelings of grief quite easily: I have permission to do *this* . . . but not to talk of my efforts to define a new life that includes the grief but is not exclusively defined by it.

I keep a diary in which my words come tumbling out, spilling onto the pages lit by my desk-lamp. My sadness takes a sturdy unyielding shape once the ink has dried on the pages:

I was playing the piano just now, when a flash of sadness and fear pulled me down. In my little wave of tears, I swam against a rip of fear. I'm fearful of how my new life is now surging ahead so strongly in a direction I never imagined, never foresaw. I'm fearful that this surge, now so fluid, might seize up and cement itself into a monolithic frieze, embalming me alive; a frieze which shows no images, shadows nor reliefs of love or children. The flow of my life has a tidal quality of unsuspecting depths and power, chillingly lonely. What if I flow along the tide so fast, so helplessly that love's hooks elude me, fail to snag on my flesh and catch me in its heartfelt embrace?

In my diary, I can emphasise, expand, or elaborate with a determination born of my drive to heat-seal my sorrow; to stop it leaking over the edges of the pages back into my life again. I toss the pain-charged words around, crossing and slashing and inserting and moving them around with a furious haste—the hastier the better—until I am quite emptied of all my hurts, sadnesses and tears. And when I have done this, I find I am surprisingly whole; I am muscular with the urge to move on to the next moment in time.

The irony is that while I am able to write freely—wantonly even—of my grief, I feel constrained in my attempts to describe or define myself as a mother-without-child because this implies a lopsidedness in me. But even though I have a space where Jack once was, this does not mean my life is half or three-quarters of a life. My life is a whole life, different certainly from the one I had planned 10 years ago, but it is still whole. And that very wholeness provides the platform for my life as mother-without-child.

I am a mother. I gave birth to a child. My child died. This does not make me 'not-a-mother'. And yet I am nervous about testing this belief beyond the simple statement of that mantra-like phrase: 'I am a mother'. The boldness of my declaration withers and fades away in my attempts to describe my meaning; to describe how it *gives* meaning to my life. I hear the words echoing without resonance: they fall with a tinny clink into the sheen of social decorum.

I am prone to physical and emotional clumsiness even at the best of times. My repeated efforts to be 'mature', to be tactful and discreet are just that—repeated efforts. My friends' patience has allowed me considerable latitude over the years. Consequently, I feel ungratefully large and oafish when I want to strain against the threads of social niceties and timidity by staking out even a little bit *more* territory for myself, to be recognised not as a 'bereaved mother' but simply as a 'mother'. I don't know how to measure my private sadness in public spaces. How do I take part in the lives and conversations of my 'mother-friends' without snagging on the pain of their embarrassed guilt at their own good luck, the bonniness of their children?

Maybe I am being too literal. Maybe I am making an issue of nothing. It's just that I feel gritty with irritation and selfconsciousness when I suspect that a friend or acquaintance is regarding me exclusively within the picture-frame of death, because it is not Jack's death which has defined me: it is Jack's birth, Jack's life, Jack's 'beingness' which has defined me.

I still remember—admittedly with a clarity now time-rubbed at the edges—details of Jack's birth: the uncomfortable grating of my left hip on the thin bed as I breathed the refrain 'every contraction is a hug and massage for the baby'; the flashpoint moment of Jack's entry, his face collapsed into bulldog folds of crossness, peering accusingly up at me. For days—possibly even for weeks—I was in tumult, replaying in my mind every whimper, shudder and roll of my body as I yielded Jack from my protective custody into an unsafe world.

And yet . . . and yet my brief life-affair with Jack was not the sunny fairytale I had blessed myself with. Like many mothers, I felt overwhelmed and frightened by the magnitude of what I had done, and set about quelling my fears by adopting a brisk, businesslike approach to the task of loving Jack, of caring for him. I fought to establish a routine. I struggled to be motherly, to be absorbed by the minutiae and tedium of milky breasts, towelling nappies and staccato conversations cut even shorter by Jack's despotic cries of hunger. I suppressed those bubbling heretic moments of boredom and worried about my initial absence of spontaneous joy. My life with Jack was knotty with bursts of powerful emotion sliding into long moments of contentment.

During Jack's brief life, I struggled to be as good a mother as I could be to him: just because he has died, I see no reason to abandon this struggle . . . and make no mistake, it has been a struggle.

I feel the hollow egg of loneliness sitting lumpishly under my heart. It is very hard to keep my motivation chugging along. I keep trying to remember how I made the effort to survive Jack's death. I can't remember where I got the energy from, how I did it.

But when Jack died, my life did not necessarily splinter neatly into two halves, with maternal joy on one side, and maternal sorrow on the other. While Jack's death has cast a shadow across my life, I do not see my days as being played out in a darker shadow of grief. Instead, as the years glide by with their own mysterious momentum, I have learned to enjoy moments of contentment that counterpoint my sorrow-driven maternal energy.

Pulling my way through the cool water
Leaving a wake as I murmur through the sheer cloth of water,
its silkiness bathing me in calm.
Muscular strokes, zig-zagging under the water, loosely etching
an arc through the air
before stretching out and pulling again.
Body rolls, rises on one side
Slicing through the blue-cream-sheer veil
Cresting
Cascading
Breathing on the stroke of three in time to my own waltz.
Swoop down to touch the wall
before turning again.
Hypnotic rhythm broken only by the occasional wheeze of
rushed breath.
Rippling water, regular strokes
Body becomes the water, dolphin-like,
Surging, undulating,

Exhilaration and calm.
Surge, slow down
Cool down.
Three more laps
Two more strokes
One last lunge to the wall.
Aah . . . swimming on a Sunday morning: a delight.

My path to such moments of contentment has not, of course, been direct nor straightforward. Often the very complexity and unpredictability of my grief was in itself overwhelming. I would feel guilty when I caught myself smiling or feeling relaxed, as though I had blasphemed in some way by not fitting the 'right' image of maternal bereavement: this, I imagined, was complete with faces etched deeply with sorrow's grooves, eyes hollow with listlessness, and bodies ebbing away into grief-ulcerating thinness.

At the very beginning, just days after Jack's death, I remember being energetic and frenetic, determined to retain Jack in my life somehow, in any way possible. I rushed around, choking up my days with activity, cramming them with events which I hoped would restore Jack, restore my mother-life to me. I was plunged into my worst moment when I realised that no amount of activity nor searching was actually going to resurrect Jack physically to me. The pain of this discovery was truly terrible.

But once this realisation started to settle in me, I began to discover new ways of coping: I sometimes ran hard in the evenings along bitumen footpaths, sweating out the pain; I took up gardening, pushing seeds into wet soil; I immersed myself in long draining hours of work and study, postponing my renewed aloneness. But most of all, I absorbed the wisdom of a friend who had lost her daughter, Amelia, at birth: 'Make your grief your friend and companion'. And I did . . . and I do.

I learned the rhythms of my sadness, and learned not to fear it so much, nor to struggle against it but simply to accommodate it into my life.

Consequently, while my loss is all the more singular and noticeable because I have not gone on to have more children, whose presence might otherwise have camouflaged Jack's absence to a certain degree, I have felt Jack by my side, growing invisibly and quietly. But how do I say this to my friends without feeling selfconscious? Without dreading their careful glances knowingly appraising me as 'not having let go'?

Of course, in the end, I don't say any of these things. I simply reflect on the strength of a mother's love—of my love—and continue to care for Jack by honouring him, by living my life as completely as possible. When I look into my mirror, I see myself as pink and rounded as ever, with my green eyes reflecting a keenness to guard Jack, to pursue my life as his mother.

SUSAN JOHNSON
This is My Life

The year that I turned 35, my arms began to feel empty. I remember a moment when I was sitting behind my lover in a car driving through France, staring at the back of his head. Everybody in the car was talking but all I was conscious of was a longing in my empty arms to form themselves into that ancient female crook and cradle a baby.

I was living in Paris then and my sixty-ish, childless painter friend Simone confirmed that this longing first struck the body. 'My own body did not need it,' she said in English without sentiment or regret. 'You must find out if yours does.'

My lover was an Italian-American who spoke heavily accented French. His character had a large dose of American schmaltz and an Italian love of drama, and inside his head screened private soaps in which he imagined himself as the war/foreign correspondent who finally settles down with a difficult but artistic Australian.

He cried easily and was terribly kind. He had thin lips and when I first kissed them I imagined myself falling into a kind of black abyss. I had separated from my English husband and left Hong Kong only a short time before and was not sure I wanted to kiss anyone.

I told him this but it only increased his ardour. It took days, weeks and months for him to convince me that his hands bore no weapons and that his fleshless lips opened into softness. With one finger I traced a line down his flesh and was surprised to find his skin tender.

Perhaps because I myself was broken I was writing a novel about hope. I lived in a large room with a tiny kitchen and a shower installed in a kind of cupboard. The room was off one of Paris's poorer streets and when I lay in bed I could clearly hear my neighbour's stream of piss hit the bowl of the toilet above me.

I tried to forget my lost husband as best I could but pain often roared in my chest. Yet paradoxically I was often exhilarated—when words rushed down my arm and out my blue pen, when I sipped a *café crème* and happened to look up at the dusty Paris sky. At times I even felt lucky.

My lover and I often talked of children even though we were virtual strangers. Once he sobbed in bed late at night when he spoke of the mutilated bodies of children he had once seen in a river in El Salvador. I held him and my room stank of our mutual terror.

I had never thought of myself as someone ever capable of having children. I thought it was what normal people did, people whose bodies and hearts and minds functioned in a way mine did not.

Most certainly this conviction arose from my first awareness that my body was not like everyone else's. My mother and I still dispute this, but I say I was aware of the hole in my chest as early as six, when I fell off a fishing wall onto rocks covered with oyster shells, and had to take off most of my clothes so my rescuers could get to the wounds.

In my memory I try to cling onto my shirt to cover the hole. Between my flattened nipples there is a large dent, as though God punched his clenched fist into me before he let me out. I already know that no other children, including my two younger brothers, have this flaw and that it somehow marks me.

I stand in the sun holding in front of me a blue Hawaiian shirt while fresh blood streams down my arms. There is blood on my legs, on my face, in my eyes, but all I am worried about is hanging onto the shirt so that no one will see how different I am, an outsider, how I am not a normal girl.

Now that my son is here I sometimes find myself

watching too carefully the flare of bones in his tiny boy's chest, on the lookout for the smallest hint of collapse.

It seemed to me that my body grew older faster than the rest of me. At 35 I sometimes still imagined myself a young girl bursting free, smashing imaginary fathers and impossible husbands and anything else which stood in my way. I was embarrassingly *unmade* on the inside, still groping on the water's edge while my same-aged friends had long ago swum away. My Paris lover once said to me that even my books were ahead of me and it was vital that I catch up.

I secretly looked upon my best friend Emma in Brisbane as a *grown-up*, with her long-time husband, her two children, her steady, everything-in-place life. She had a proper house, a car, living room furniture: she knew what she would be doing from one month to the next.

I thought of women who had given birth as having passed through one of life's most crucial doors, mothers somehow rendered unable to reveal the secrets they had found on the other side to those non-mothers who had not passed through.

The year I turned 35 I began to sense clumsily that I must find a way to move forward into the second half of my life, to find a way to grow up properly. I did not know if the best way of doing this was by having a child, I only knew that I had come to the end of myself. It was clear even to me that the old way of being myself was no longer working and that unless I wanted to spend the rest of my life emotionally atrophied I had better act.

When I married my first husband on a rainy day in London, my lips trembled. I had starved myself the month before and had practised saying the registry office words over and over. I thought they would halt in my mouth on the day but they came out entirely whole.

Afterwards we went to a swank London hotel with my best friend Emma's English aunt and cousins. Emma's aunt, a psychotherapist by profession, had already tried to warn me off marrying someone I had known only three months, but I thought she was jealous of our bliss, unhappy in her own dead marriage.

I had already had a bad falling out with another friend in Australia who had written to suggest that we have the honeymoon without getting married. *How dare you*, I wrote back, *have I ever told you how to run your life?*

I was so convinced I was doing the right thing I would have killed anyone who had tried to stop me. All my instincts were telling me it was right, every nerve and muscle and fibre in my body screamed out that my husband was going to be my husband for the rest of my life.

In Hong Kong six months later a voice inside me tried to announce I had been wrong. I immediately stilled it but was instantly flooded with shame, horrified by what was to come.

If my own instincts were wrong, how could I trust anything again?

My husband and I had quickly spoken of babies. We had identically crooked eye teeth and the very first night we had dinner together in Paris we joked that so would our children.

I was 32 then, and in reality having children seemed to me a long way off, in reality I suffered a kind of psychic terror every time I thought seriously of it. It seemed to me that whatever I was made of was not strong enough to bear it, either physically or emotionally.

I was not yet ready either to relinquish the stage, to gladly pass the torch to those coming up from behind. If secretly I felt I could not yet handle the responsibility of children, I also felt a mean-spirited urge to keep hogging the light. My life was still unfurling, I was still having trouble imagining myself fully grown, let alone imagining someone else's growing.

In short, I was remarkably self-centred, emotionally stranded somewhere around adolescence. Is it any wonder that my marriage began to fall apart around my head, that my husband and I began to squabble like the children we were?

Some readers (and the occasional friend) think of my

novels as my life served up reheated but I know my actual life is not shaped like fiction at all. My books are my means of ordering the world to attention: in real life husbands never go in the direction I want them to go and I can never see well enough in the gloom.

At some point after I left my husband I slunk back to Australia. If I had been able I would have told no one of my return and never set foot outside the door, so total was my sense of humiliation. For the first time in my life I felt that I was fundamentally broken and might never heal, that whatever old tricks I had used before to get myself to stand up again were no longer of any use.

Amazingly, I kept writing the novel about hope while all hope inside me was extinguished. While I felt my old self to be effectively dead I kept doggedly writing about a boy whose hopeful innocence saved him.

At some point I went back to Paris again and took up with the Italian-American lover who tried to convince me I was not dead. I believe his own grief was attracted to mine and that he thought he could save me.

Sometimes now when I look at my son I still wonder how he got here. He has survived his first year as he survived his birth and marvellous conception.

I will never forget the night he came home when a fire

burned in the street below. I can still feel my naked feet standing on the small concrete verandah eight storeys up, watching the people milling in the street below, watching the night sky, the spasmodic red flash of fire engine lights. The whole world appeared struck by catastrophe.

As I stood there I was seized by panic: my heart began to palpitate wildly. I stood feeling my feet on the concrete, immobilised by terror, amazed that neither my husband nor my mother could see my fear.

I inched my way back inside and sat down on the couch, consciously trying to slow my breathing. I had once learned a Buddhist meditation practice and I practised it then, feeling the ordinary world only slowly returning to me.

And then the baby cried and suddenly I was no longer frightened. By the time I picked him up I had the strangest sensation that my son was pulling calmness from me, that his requirements had somehow forced me to quell my own anxiety. It was the first lesson my son taught me.

For if considering whether to have a child is all about oneself, the arrival of the actual child extinguishes everything but the child. A baby obliterates the known world, reducing the scale of the entire universe to its own four limbs.

If I wanted to be taken up and used in a way I had never been before, then surely I was. Everything I had known was of no use to me and for the first time in my life I had to give up my long-cherished conviction that Effort Equals Outcome.

Caspar was and is the wild card in my game of life, the ultimate Zen test for this perfectionist. I do things and can never be sure of the result, whether it's to do with his sleeping, his eating, or his smile.

He obviously came to earth to teach me some things. The biggest and best lesson is this: life is not exclusively about myself anymore.

But before he arrived I continued in that dreamy state of believing that having a baby was mostly about me. All through my pregnancy I monitored how I was feeling and continued to harbour private qualms about something going wrong.

I had suffered a miscarriage only months before and expected blood every time I looked down. I did not know how my fixed-up chest with its scar and steel pin would cope with my expanding uterus and one night I dreamed that my scar burst open.

The doctor in London reassured me that the operation I had had at 16, in which my breastbone was broken and re-set with a steel pin, could easily withstand a growing uterus beneath it holding a kicking baby. I was still not convinced, for I had long ceased to think of my body as normal.

At night my chest hurt beneath my ribs and my new husband lay fresh hot flannels against my skin to ease the pain. Both of us knew without the need of tests that our baby was a boy but only I secretly doubted whether my outsider's body could produce something whole.

I no longer remember the exact steps I took in my growing-up journey. I know only that it had something to do with the collapse of my first marriage and the great jolt that gave me, along with the kindness of my Italian-American lover, even though I subsequently learned that he loved me best when I was grief-stricken and far away and that when I turned my face towards him he grew afraid.

It had to do, too, with long nights by myself where I stared down my own aloneness and dared imagine that I might be growing old. Somehow I began to feel that I had passed through barren land to end up in a place where I was comfortable enough to invite other people (even a baby) in.

By the time I met in London the Australian man who was to become my second husband, I felt both larger and smaller, calmer and certainly humbler. I no longer saw my life as an endless vista, opening eternally before me.

A woman friend of roughly the same age as me had died of AIDS contracted through heterosexual sex, and I had gone through a crazy time of projecting my inner fears onto something outer, even convincing myself at one stage that I had contracted AIDS too, no matter how many tests I had which proved otherwise, no matter how much a small rational part of me knew I was being wildly irrational. Yet somehow I managed to come out the other side, finally able to experience myself as a fully-grown, middle-aged woman.

By the time I met my second husband I was ready for a baby and to my surprise, at 37, my body agreed.

Our son Caspar was born at 3.59 in Sydney on a Tuesday winter afternoon. It was the most powerful, *convulsive* act of my life. Just before he emerged from my body he turned around and I felt my internal organs convulse with an enormous energy. I felt the hand of God squeezing the life from me; I was spastic with it, possessed, and then I felt a quietness come and I stopped moaning and started to breathe and Caspar's head came out into the water, and with the next push the midwife's hands brought the rest of him up to break the surface.

As soon as I saw him I knew he was mine, the baby I had taken so long to grow up for. I turned around in the bath to look at Les, shouting, 'He's here, Les, Caspar's here!' The baby was crying and so was I and I think Les was too although he was also laughing.

I could not believe all the joy my arms held, that my arms knew exactly how to hold him. In one stroke I had joined the world, became a member of the older generation and for the first time knew myself to be an ordinary woman.

Reader, this is no story. Reader, This Is My Life.

KARINA KELLY
Living in Colour

More. That's how I'd describe parenthood. More exhausting, more frustrating and more wonderful than I could possibly have imagined. It's as though I had walked through a gateway from a small enclosed garden out into the wild and wide expanse of nature.

I didn't just fall into motherhood. I first had to be convinced that I wanted to be there. How could something that happens to millions of women every day be so special? I watched my friends with children, and didn't get clucky. Snotty-nosed children with sticky fingers trying to monopolise their parents who invariably claimed, 'I don't know what's got into him—he's not usually like this'. I heard tales of sleepless nights, of tantrums, of illness and dirty nappies. I studied their faces carefully. There were dark bags under their eyes, more grey hairs and wrinkles than in their child-free days only a year or two before.

Yet, despite the constant moaning about never seeing a movie, despite describing sleep as a hungry person speaks about food, they had a strange air of satisfaction about them—especially the mothers. I couldn't put my finger on it. What was that look? It seemed ridiculous but I'd swear it was smugness. What on earth did they have to feel smug about? And after the complaints, there was always the disclaimer: 'But I'd never go back to life without her'; 'We wouldn't have it any other way'. In my uncharitable moments, I wondered if my friends were all conspiring to say parenthood was wonderful so that I would be encouraged enough to join them in their suffering.

The only thing that I did know is that parenthood is irrevocable. Houses and even husbands and wives can be changed but your children—they're yours until death do you part. Were we ready for that responsibility? Is one ever?

Then, as my 30th birthday came and went I softened to the idea. But for all the wrong reasons. I thought it would be wonderful to have a child who we could pass our thoughts on to, who would come to share our values and views on the world. It was for almost academic reasons that I thought it would be good to have a child. Then I didn't get pregnant for a long, long time—over two years. So by the time I did, I'd made a significant journey from serious doubt to a sense of achievement at just being pregnant.

We named my bump Sproglett, and took it off to have an ultrasound. As soon as the image came up, there was Sproglett with its hands up over its ears. Now, the doctors tell me that foetuses can't hear ultrasounds—so maybe Sproglett had some other reason for putting its hands over its ears—perhaps my stomach was overactive that day. But, as any parent will tell you (and yes, we are all conspiring), that first image of your baby at 16 weeks' gestation makes the pregnancy feel more real. The images produced should be on page one of your baby photo album.

I read voraciously. Every book about pregnancy I could get my hands on. I became an authority on every potential obscure complication and problem. I knew the odds of complications were low, but the sheer number of possibilities (and the fact that the information was taking up such a large amount of space in my brain) seemed to magnify the risks.

'It's a girl,' said the obstetrician's secretary. 'I can tell from your shape.' And this female chauvinism continued throughout my pregnancy.

'How do you feel?'

'Fantastic,' I would reply. 'I wish I could feel like this all the time!'

'It must be a girl,' they'd whisper. 'Does it kick much?'

'No, hardly feel a thing.'

'Ah, then it's a girl.' My husband, David, was the only one who thought it would be a boy.

I was astounded by how political childbirth is. On one side, there's the male-dominated obstetrics profession, offering every latest medical intervention. On the other, the midwives, appealing to mothers-to-be to have a natural childbirth, and in the process, wresting women's bodies back from male doctors and male-dominated science. While the natural birth option appealed, I also knew that, male-dominated or not, science had things to teach us. And you don't need to read a lot of history to know how many women used to die in childbirth. I decided to take a middle course and I found myself a female obstetrician who had had three children herself. No doctor was going to tell me that I 'might experience some discomfort' during childbirth. She didn't.

I wrote a birth plan which was a complete waste of time. I think it said something like 'prefer not to have epidural'. The due date came and went. As it turned out I had the longest induction in the history of the world. Forty-eight hours it took, but for the first 24, nothing happened; then, after 18 hours of contractions and no sleep I began to understand how people might feel when they are being tortured. In the hospital ward we were several storeys up. I remember analysing the catches on the windows carefully. I remember seriously considering throwing myself out. Then, after yet another go in the hot tub—which worked well to ease the pain but made me wonder if I would give birth to an already-cooked lobster—they examined me and told me I was two centimetres dilated. What does this mean? If you were on a train trip from Sydney to Melbourne, you'd just be leaving the platform at Central Station.

This baby just didn't want to get born. At this point I became seriously discouraged. Time seemed to be standing still. When the doors swung open, I could hear the screams of the other women giving birth on either side of me. I seemed unable to scream. I tried moaning a bit but it just made me feel depressed as well as in pain. Here I was, trapped in some weird time warp, trying to give birth while babies were being born in rooms on either side of me. The women and their babies went home. The babies grew up and went to university and I was still in that birthing room waiting for the baby that wouldn't come out.

'I want an epidural,' I said, trying not to sound emotional.

David said, 'You don't want an epidural.'

'Yes I do,' I said, as women by the thousands had said before me. What a blessed relief it was, too. After the epidural, my mother, Irene, read me the next three days' menus and ticked them off for me. Of course, my mother never had the choice of an epidural. In fact when I asked her to be present at the birth, she wasn't sure if she wanted to see me in such distress. I still had another six hours before the baby was born—after a weaker top-up of epidural I was able to push with the contractions and when the baby was finally born it was without intervention.

As soon as the head crowned, the baby changed tactics. Suddenly, instead of dawdling, this baby was in a hurry. It shot out so fast the doctor nearly dropped it. They set up a mirror so that I too could see the baby being born. It was an amazing sight.

My goodness, it's a boy! And look at that cleft chin! Every muscle in his tiny face was working overtime. It was like he was going through every emotion there is, in fast forward. Because he was overdue, he had no vernix on him. He didn't look like a tiny cross-Channel swimmer covered in white grease. He was just shiny and pink and of course the most beautiful baby I had ever clapped eyes on. My mother was now very glad that she had come. Despite having had three children herself, she'd never witnessed a birth. My baby was on the breast within half an hour—I didn't have to teach him anything. That should have given me an inkling of what was to come.

Like most mothers used to being organised professionals, I underestimated how much work a baby would be. We named our baby Adam and for the first two weeks he wore a worried expression on his face. The spots where his eyebrows would one day be were pulled together in apprehension. I think the birth had been just as traumatic for him as for me. After 14 days I think he came to the conclusion that this strange world full of loud noises, bright lights and new smells was not so bad after all, and he relaxed. He doubled his weight in only seven weeks and because he was totally bald, was now a contender to be the Michelin Baby. I still remember the moment many months later when I kissed the top of his head and felt more than just bare skin.

As time went on I was rather peeved to discover that Adam was more relaxed and playful with David or my mother. When I came near he started panting and poking his tongue out, pushing the surface of his tongue against his top lip as if he were tasting ice cream. So it had come to this—I was just a sex object to this little creature!

The birth plan may have been a waste of time but keeping a journal wasn't. I now look back on this with great pleasure. Each time I dip into it, I relive the strong feelings I had at the time and recall details that have faded from my memory. At six-and-a-half weeks, David and I both experienced a beautiful smile. I am sure I was wandering around with that same smug, self-satisfied look I'd seen on other mothers' faces.

I'm a great believer in ceremonies and don't see why people who are not religious shouldn't enjoy them. So we organised a naming ceremony and a dear friend, Faith Bandler—who had also married us—named Adam and we all enjoyed a beautiful breakfast in the back garden. Breakfast seemed to be the only meal I was capable of organising, and I had the advantage of being up so much earlier than the guests!

It's not until you have a child that you truly experience unconditional love. No matter what this child does, you know you will be there for them. It's not until you have a child that you truly worry. If anything was to happen to that child ... well it doesn't bear thinking about. But you do. You have nightmares about it, too. And at least for me, it wasn't until I had a child that I became responsible. In fact, I think we all remain in a strange state of preserved adolescence until we are swept out of it by the daunting responsibility of parenthood.

My mother has always said that her recollection of having three young children was never finishing a sentence. It's true that life after children is fragmented. Tasks get done incrementally. Sometimes they simply don't get done. I guess my journal reflects that, too.

Adam hasn't taken to Farex like other babies. He tasted it a couple of times and has now refused point blank to eat it. When we go out to cafés Adam comes in his stroller and although at five months he doesn't eat much, we give him some bread to suck and he's happy. Today there was no plain bread—just garlic bread. So I gave that to Adam. He stuffed it into his mouth. There was a pause and then he looked as though he had just had a religious revelation. 'I have seen the Lord, and he cooks with garlic!' I could hear him think. 'So, that's what food is supposed to taste like!? You've been keeping it from me—trying to fob me off with that Farex—bah!'

. . .

Went to visit Adam at childcare today. I picked him up and sat down with him on my lap. He vomited on me with such force that I was stunned for a few seconds. It was as though someone had just poured a litre carton of custard all over me. I'd heard of projectile vomiting but until now have never experienced it first hand. I looked around helplessly. One of the carers took Adam and pointed me in the direction of the childcare centre shower. But what was I going to change into? I had to go back to the office. Did they have any spare clothes? No. Except . . . er . . . the children's dressing-up clothes. I returned to work somewhat overdressed wearing a fairy princess pink flouncy skirt and a green satin top. One of my colleagues looked up from his laptop and commented dryly, 'That's a new look for you isn't it, Karina?'

I remember things like this: that aggravating phase that children go through where they drop things all the time and wait (or yell) for you to pick them up. At the time it seems like bloody-mindedness on their part. But it occurs to me that it might be their first experiment we're witnessing. How do they know that something close looks bigger than when it's far away? I was watching a program about how hard it is to teach this to computers, when it dawned on me that this is what Adam was doing when he was dropping things and watching them so intensely. It's a part of our perception that has to be programmed in!

And then, I had no idea how funny having a child would be. Adam makes me laugh every day. Despite the responsibility and tiredness and frustration, I find the observations he makes a constant delight. It breaks down all that cynicism and world-weariness, built up in my brain over the years like the scunge on the inside of a kettle.

I suppose the humour stems from simply seeing the world through the eyes of an alien. Not knowing the correct words, Adam would make them up. A helium balloon was an 'up-ball', David's morning stubble was 'grass on face'. Later it was animal mania, perhaps because we often visit the zoo, and a local park where we feed the ducks.

We've been to our favourite Chinese restaurant where we ordered duck. When the steaming plate arrived Adam carefully described what he thought must be the process. 'You go to the park,' he said, 'and you pick up a duck and you put it in the oven and you turn it into meat.' Why did we find that so hilariously funny? Because we don't like to think about the fact that we eat animals, and have done our best to separate the animals we socialise with from the ones we eat.

Later for dessert, I ask Adam if he would like to have

ice-cream with caramel sauce. He looks surprised, but says yes. When it arrives he asks if this is the camel sauce. Certainly it's the right colour. After the meal we tell him we have to wait for the bill. But for him instead, we're 'waiting for the bilby'.

Adam's development of humour has also made me think about the nature of humour itself. We start off with jokes like, 'What are hundreds and thousands?—Smarties poo!' In fact all that poo and bum stuff, which I always thought was just because little children went through a smutty stage, has a reason for being there. One of the hardest things for young children to learn is the control of their bladders and bowels. They know where it 'should' go. It may well be their strongest and most formative social convention. So *not* doing it where it should be done is as funny to them as Elle McFeast or Basil Fawlty are to us. The only difference is that the social conventions that are being flouted are a bit more complex in the adult version.

Trying to understand society's conventions is difficult, but we're working on the subtleties. We have discussed whether kangaroos can talk, what actually constitutes 'naughtiness', where the sun goes when it goes down and how plants 'have a drink' when it rains. One of the most alarming concepts has been pregnancy. When Adam was two-and-a-half we explained that a friend had a baby in her tummy. We showed him pictures of me when I was pregnant and explained that he had also once been in my tummy. He looked absolutely aghast and turned to me and said, 'Mummy—did you eat me?'

These days with Adam nearly five, we've left the elementary stuff behind. The next bit of software development will take about 20 years. He's starting school in a few months. A friend at the ABC told me a story about his child starting school. His parents had told him frequently that he would be going to school soon. 'When do I stop school?' he had asked. He was told, 'When you are eighteen.' The child became increasingly agitated until the first day of school. He turned anxiously to his mother and said, 'Will you come and get me when I'm eighteen?'

Of course we also do so much for our children because we see them as an extension of ourselves. They are our immortality. For most of us, they will be the most enduring and impressive legacy we leave on this earth. Adam has taught me how to share and give and how to love unconditionally. He has shown me that I can be much more than I was before. It's as though before he came along I was living my life in black and white and now I'm living in colour.

TRISHA GODDARD
A Tale of Two Pregnancies

My first experience with any human being under the age of your average *Play School* fan, was when visiting my dearest darling friend, Clarrie, after the birth of Sam. Clarrie, let me explain, is my kind of woman. Together, witty, go-getting, beautiful, vulnerable but very, very ballsy.

So I stood there, by her hospital bed, only just visible above a jungle of bouquets, a very worried mate. She insisted on giving me a running commentary about the meconium that her baby son was red-facedly squeezing out of his bum. That was it. The old Clarrie was gone. Finished. This was a Stepford wife thing who'd never get pissed again, never bitch about bitches again, never be wild again.

I held Sam once in my arms, when later Clarrie visited

me, my face aching from bunging on this 'what a lovely baby' smile from the minute she walked in the door. Her voice was softer than it used to be. Her movements were all 'Johnson & Johnson'—in fact she had gone all soft-focus on me. The scariest thing was that she was acting as if this was normal.

And lo! I joined the ranks of all the fools who have ever uttered those famous last words: 'I'll never let any baby change *my* lifestyle.'

Fast forward 18 months to about the third stupid pregnancy kit that insisted I *was* pregnant. I know Capricorns are meant to be cynical, but I was ready to sue the chemist. I was actually surprised when my doctor confirmed the result, even though I had been trying to get pregnant at the time! There was still that 'but surely, this can't be happening to me' foolishness going on. Thankfully, when I stared at myself in the mirror, there wasn't a hint of soft-focus about me. I was not going to be replaced by a 'Nappy Ad' version of myself. I was going to fight to stay ME!

I was fronting the New South Wales 7.30 *Report* on the ABC at the time. It was a very blokey period in news and current affairs and I was determined I could carry on in the pseudo-blokey way that was pretty much the unspoken rule. I went to ridiculous lengths. If I was offered a chair, I made a great point of glaring at the offerer as if I'd been insulted. I approached pregnancy in an investigative way that would have put Chris Masters to

shame. However, I never discussed any of my research
with my colleagues, and little did they know that I knew
exactly what was happening inside my body at any given
moment.

I would start the day at seven am jumping around the
studios, for the taping of a *Play School* program, singing
and dancing like it was the normal thing every woman
did heading for the seventh month of pregnancy. Finish
at 12. Lie down and meditate in a dark room for 20
minutes. Then go upstairs and start work on the *7.30
Report*. Go live to air that evening and drive home at
eight o'clock so exhausted that the 10-minute drive would
take me half an hour, as I'd keep falling asleep at the
wheel and keep having to pull over.

And all this time I was working out in the gym about
five times a week. Not a drop of alcohol touched my lips
because I was in training, buddy. I actually used to get
off on watching the looks of amazement as I did stuff that
many of the unpregnant couldn't. You see, I was brought
up in East Africa where childbirth had never been
eulogised by an advertising agency. Women simply worked
in the fields, got pregnant, had their babies and went
back to hoeing the row. No fluffy slippers, no flowers and
certainly no being treated as if they might fall apart like
eggshells at any moment.

I liked their approach. It was going to be mine. I figured
early on in the piece that since I had learned to work
with—in fact welcome—the pain I went through in the

gym, I could do it in childbirth. I figured if I had 10 children, 10 evil sessions of torturous labour lasting 24 hours each, that would still only be 10 days out of my life. Big deal!

At least I'd be sure to lose weight at the end of it, which was more than I could say for the workouts I was doing.

The media seemed absolutely fascinated with the idea that a woman could be pregnant and . . . well, what? Hold it together enough to read an autocue or do an interview? Journalists kept asking me for funny anecdotes about being a pregnant TV person. I think their encouraging smiles were more expectant than I felt. They kept writing stories with the word 'Super' in it. 'Superfit', 'Supermum' . . . I think I become a sort of hero to workaholic females. You know, 'How to fit baby in between your daily workout and first conference call.'

All of a sudden, I was no longer 'Trish' around the ABC corridors. I was suddenly 'Mum'. That drove me wild! I had about as much mothering instinct as any of my other career-driven, single macho colleagues.

I *did* my first pregnancy. You know, like someone *does* a degree. I was intensely interested in what was going on inside me, but I felt totally detached. Emotionally, I kept myself very isolated—from my partner, from everyone, even from dearest Clarrie. Don't get me wrong, I wasn't depressed, rather just not *impressed*. I don't think my colleagues knew quite how to treat me. I think they ended up ignoring my pregnancy as much as I seemed to, although one of my producers (who was also a mate) blamed my partner for ruining my life.

I researched how blossoming mothers were meant to behave and played that role when appropriate—in supermarkets near the baby goods aisle. I kept reading all this stuff about bonding with the baby, but the only time I really felt this baby existed was when it kicked the hell out of me while I was trying to read an intro live on air. Try keeping a straight face when someone is playing interuterine Nintendo! But I got used to that too. I didn't *hate* my baby. I didn't really *anything* it.

I was disgustingly fit. Not a day's nausea ... except when one of those baby ads came on TV. I had by now turned into a Total Teetotaller Fitness Fascist. There is, somewhere, a plaque dedicated to the memory of some poor fool who got into a lift with me while puffing on a cigarette (this was in the pre no-smoking in the workplace days). I treated him in the same way one would for the crime of infanticide. While friends quaffed wine, I sat there smiling at them in much the same way Joan of Arc would have stared out of the flames.

I think I actually enjoyed all the denial stuff. This baby was going to get the best damned start ever. If I could do without alcohol a few years back when working in Saudi Arabia and all for the mighty dollar, surely I could do without alcohol for the sake of a human life, I reasoned. And surely, my bloody partner could support me by also abstaining. I will recount his reaction in my memoirs under the title, 'How To Absolutely Terrify the Average Australian Male'. If I haven't mentioned my then partner until now, it's because in my mind, as with most men, he was pretty shut out of the whole process, except when I insisted he read up on each stage I was experiencing.

I think the only time I felt vulnerable was when my partner was away and an English mate of mine was staying with me. She was rather prone to hysterics and when I awoke one morning with an excruciating and very worrying pain in my back, I literally dragged myself around the flat in order not to wake her up. I didn't feel like a Tosca type drama, I felt like death. My doctor decided I should call an ambulance and go straight to hospital. No way José! I ordered a cab and dragged myself into it, barking at the driver not to be so bloody stupid. There was no way I was going to give birth (if that's what the pain was) on a vinyl seat when I had specially taken out private health insurance. When I got to the hospital, they put me in a wheelchair and took me via underground corridors to the maternity unit admission. It was there that a few people started to recognise me and point and whisper. In total agony, and by now in tears, for the first time worrying about 'the baby', I called a nurse over.

'Can't I wait somewhere else?' I sobbed. 'Those people are all looking at me.'

'That's no problem,' she said, and promptly turned my wheelchair around so that I was facing the wall.

That experience set the tone for the rest of that awful morning. The hanging about for someone to come and see me became more painful than the pinched nerve in my back. Besides, the baby was shifting its position much faster than the overworked doctors were shifting theirs. So I promptly discharged myself and got a cab home, the dire warnings of nurses ringing in my ears.

My Pommie house guest did a total Tosca as to why I hadn't awoken her at the beginning of Act One.

During my pregnancy, my GP had recommended that I go to prenatal classes held by one JuJu Sundin, which I did. I also went to classes held for mothers and fathers-to-be at a local public hospital. While the sweet midwife there talked about breathing and relaxation, JuJu Sundin was totally outrageous. 'This is big pain we're talking about,' she said. 'You need big ways to cope with it!' She had us waddly ones shouting, making childbirth noises at the top of our voices—grunts for some, orgasmic-type screams for those who'd forgotten what got them into this mess in the first place. She told us about releasing endorphins and going with the flow, demanding and getting what we wanted—real empowering stuff. *This* was far more African than ad agency, I thought. I like this.

Billie was born two weeks early. I put it down to shock. Two nights before she was born, my partner was interstate. I staggered out to put the rubbish bins in the street for the next day's collection. There was a car on the opposite side of the road. With near panic I realised that the occupants were watching me. Suddenly, one of them came out of the car and walked towards me. 'Here, let me help with that,' he said. In case you think I was having a bout of pregnancy-induced paranoia, let me point out that this apparent knight in the night had a couple of cameras swinging from his neck.

'No it's OK. Who are you anyway?' I asked, my heart thumping and my body stupidly getting into flight or fight mode (more like stumble and rumble mode when you're almost nine months gone).

'Oh, I'm a photographer from the *Sun*,' he said. 'We're staking out your place 'cos we heard you'd be having your baby any minute and we wanted to get a picture of you going off to hospital.'

I fled back inside at about 30 waddles per minute and spent the rest of the evening alternating between anger and fear. A couple of hours after I finally fell asleep, I was rudely awakened by the doorbell. There was a smartly dressed young woman from a rival newspaper with a photographer who wanted the same thing as the previous hack. I stood there, blinking in my oversize Mickey Mouse T-shirt, hair that would be the pride of any punk-rocker, as the photographer tried to get a shot of me through the door . . . luckily for my image, without success. But I was really rattled.

I don't think it any coincidence that I had what felt like an upset tummy that night when my partner returned. It continued into the morning and I started to get a bit suspicious. I stopped listening to all the radio news and current affairs and rang up dear Clarrie and asked her to describe what early labour pains felt like. Halfway through her description I got a huge cramp and automatically started panting as I listened to her. 'Er,' she said, '*that's* exactly what they sound like! You're in labour. You'd better go to hospital.'

I wasn't going without breakfast. Decided on fresh mango and insisted my partner stop at the local newsagent on the way to the hospital, just in case this was a false alarm and I found myself on air at 7.30 that night without a clue as to what was happening in the world. And that's how I was driven to hospital. Reading the papers and researching. I started taking things seriously about five minutes away from the hospital, mainly because the contractions were starting to get pretty serious themselves and my reading kept being interrupted. It was getting to me. It hurt. Bad!

As I walked into the hospital foyer, a group of schoolchildren led by a teacher walked past me. Lo and behold, the first full force contraction hit me like a sledgehammer. I remembered what I'd learned from my childbirth guru, JuJu Sundin. This was mega pain and called for mega action. So right there and then I leaned against a wall, and stamped and roared like a rhinoceros on heat.

I vaguely remember hearing, 'But, miss, that's the lady from *Play School*. What's she doing?' In the middle of everything I managed a laugh. Boy, did that teacher have her afternoon's work cut out for her!

That laugh lightened me up. Hey, this pain was great! It meant things were happening. Every contraction brought me closer to that exciting moment when I'd at last get to see this thing. I was introducing a new life to this planet. Such a monumental step, such passage from girl to real woman, had to be a unique experience. I embraced my pain. I had such a positive view of it. I welcomed each contraction with, 'Great! The baby's moving, turning, going down!' I've since learned that telling people you enjoyed childbirth is like telling people you like snuff films . . . you're likely to be seen as a sicko.

I roared, chanted, bashed my partner in the groin, put on heavy street funk music, took it off and put on Tommy Emmanuel and Vince Jones, threw up the mango breakfast and didn't bother with any of the painkillers.

Two-and-a-half hours later after one orgasmic, sensational push, Billie was born. My obstetrician, partner and I all counted her fingers and toes together like a feverish kindergarten class. I was on a high. When the nurse read out the time of birth I suddenly realised I had forgotten to call work! There was a phone above the bed I'd been cavorting around and squatting on, and I called the office as the nurses were working out Billie's APGAR score.

I talked to my executive producer. 'Deb,' I started, 'er . . . I don't think I'll be coming in. You see . . . ' And right on cue, Billie wailed. Deb didn't miss a beat. 'Can we get a crew down there?' I didn't miss a beat either. This would be a way of killing all the other press interest. 'Yeah,' I said in my best 'Blokese'. 'Here's the deal. Mark [my partner] will produce it, no extra footage. I'll do a piece to camera to top and tail the show. Get hold of the make-up department and have the crew bring some stuff over.'

I cuddled my baby, got off the bed, had a shower, got fully and smartly dressed and made-up, and two hours after Billie was born, I topped and tailed that evening's *7.30 Report*. Absolutely bloody mad! But I was on a high and the bosses went all new age about it. And it rated its milk-laden tits off.

I had Billie on the Thursday, left hospital on the following Wednesday, dropped by home and then went straight to the studio to do the show with the baby. In those days we used three camera people, so the rule was that whoever wasn't actually shooting, held the baby. And so, hip young grooves and surly blokes cradled my baby through the show. I got curtains in the office and breastfed. I think most people were too bound up by the laws of (up till then theoretical) political correctness to be too overt in their reactions to all this. But they got used to it because I breastfed Billie for 18 months and we both absolutely adored it.

So cut to pregnancy number two, four years later. By this stage at 36 I was finding the prospect of another fat tummy in TV-image land all a bit of a challenge. But I finally bit the bullet and did it. I'd read the research about single children and decided there was no way Billie was going to be one.

This pregnancy was completely different. I didn't just have morning sickness, I had midday sickness, afternoon sickness, evening and night sickness—for five months. I didn't whinge about it. I accepted it on a day by day basis. I still wasn't drinking, but I was far less fanatical about the whole thing—in other words, those around me were allowed to throw their health to the wind and I didn't lecture them or martyr myself.

Unfortunately though, I was working even harder than when I was at the ABC. This time I was part-owner, producer, and major philosophy behind a daily health chat show on Channel Ten, called *Live It Up*. I was boss, presenter, writer, mother hen to staff, the lot . . . and unknown to me I was running on empty and burning out fast. I was power walking for an hour about six times a week and I had a fantastic personal trainer, Craig, who taught me boxing. Under his supervision I was pushing weights I never had before.

I began to understand those stories of how the Eastern Bloc coaches used to get young female athletes pregnant and make them abort the baby at three months. Sick, but they recognised how women become so much stronger and more flexible when pregnant. I loved my training sessions. In a society that designs fragile-looking virginal maternity outfits for the one time in your life that you're shouting from the rooftops that you've had at least one bonk, it was great being tough and strong.

When my husband suggested going to Western Australia for the Christmas holidays so I could finally get to see him surf and drive him from winery to winery in Margaret River, my answer resembled that famous vomit scene in *The Exorcist*. Instead, I went off to England to see mummy and daddy with Billie, because when you are pregnant, you need your mummy and daddy.

While I was in England and could relax, I realised how much my sickness had made me feel fragile and vulnerable. Despite the fact that I could probably lift a 10 tonne truck, I couldn't lift the feeling of dread even after I got back to Australia. But I had set a precedent in the 'I can do it all by myself' department and besides, unknown to me, my husband was having an affair. The result was total emotional isolation and fear, though at the time I didn't know about what. My feeling of danger just around the corner was so monumental that I actually went to see a psychologist, trying to understand why I was prepared to talk about everything but what my husband thought about what was going on. In hindsight, I understood.

I talk about this because I have had numerous letters, heard numerous anecdotes, about men who have affairs when their wives are pregnant. But it's something no one wants to talk about, even though it happens so often. No one wants to shatter that ad agency, soft-focus image of pregnant woman being cuddled and protected by involved, loving, supportive man. It's too scary for women to think about, and too guilt provoking for men to want to face. But I wish we would. All that time I couldn't understand why my husband refused to put his hand on my tummy when the baby kicked. It was about his guilt, not about our baby.

I have virtually wiped the memory of my second pregnancy from my soul. It is too painful to remember. But I do remember constantly talking to Billie about Madison while I was pregnant. I'd known I was having a girl and she'd been named as soon as we knew. Billie and I would daydream about Madi. When I had been pregnant with Billie, her constant fluttery kicks and hiccoughs had given me some intuitive insight to her personality . . . like a nervous, pretty, excited little butterfly. Likewise I knew from Madi's get-you-in-the-guts kicks that she was going to be a slow and solid truck. Mothers-to-be, trust your intuition—I was right!

If I was fit for Billie's birth, I was ultra fit, physically, at least, for Madi's birth. This time, she was two weeks late and I had to have my waters broken to get her out. Again typical of her character. Billie always rushes ahead without a care in the world. Madi is slow, stubborn, takes in all the possibilities and deliberately lags behind.

I had no painkillers, a two-hour, forty-five minute labour this time. Had Madi on the Thursday, did a one-hour power walk on the Friday and Saturday and went home on the Sunday. I was back at work on Monday and back on screen by Wednesday, breastfeeding between shows. I just kept going. Not quite like last time, though, because this time I didn't want to play the bloke. I was boss lady now, I didn't have to—at least in theory. In reality the hub of my company's business was my moniker on screen. I couldn't get off the roundabout even if the ride was making me sick.

The next 12 weeks were the worst of my life. When my baby was seven weeks old, I nearly lost her. She lay in hospital surrounded by tubes because of a life-threatening illness. I prayed and did deals with God and slept on a mattress on the floor by her cot, existing in a suspended state of panic for five days. Five weeks later, I finally found out about my husband's affair—with someone I knew very well and trusted. It had been going on since I was six months pregnant. My planet fell apart when it was at its weakest anyway.

I spent the next four weeks breastfeeding my darling Madi in a psychiatric unit.

But there is a happy ending. I've been a single mother since Madi was 12 weeks old and Billie was almost five, and I agree with recent UK research that shows that in spite of hard work and tough times (or maybe because), single mothers have more pride, more of a sense of achievement and more satisfaction than their married counterparts. We also tend to be closer to our children.

I have learned that doing it all is not about being a Supermum, it's usually about being super scared to get off the career-a-round (usually with good reason). It's also about being trapped between 1970s feminist rhetoric and 1990s soul-searching, and it's often about clinging to what you know best—being in control, and survival. For the first time in my life I am living and truly loving.

I have learned to feel sorry for the old me and all those others who utter those famous last words: 'I'll never let any baby change *my* lifestyle.'

Mind you my darling Clarrie and I still get pissed, play up, and have a laugh at both the Stepford wives and the Supermums!

LEONIE STEVENS
Mother Superior and the Kid from Hell

I was cool with this motherhood thing. People told me, Kelly, you've got no idea how much this will change your life. You just can't begin to imagine. So many people told me this so many times that my only course of action was to surrender: sit back and wait for the inevitable.

And I was cool with that. I knew I'd be okay, and Zac would probably be okay, and Leila was in fine form at her last ultrasound. She kicked and moved so much it was tricky to snap her photo.

I was calm, you see. This parenthood trip wasn't going to faze me.

Until . . .

Grace descended on the house like one of those dust clouds from out west. She was carrying a backpack of clothes, a basket of food, a bucket of Lego and the toddler from hell.

'I heard you're pregnant!' she boomed, hugging me. 'Congratulations!'

And it wasn't bad for a moment, this conspiratorial maternal hug thing, until Reptar, who was squashed between us, gave me an almighty jab to the breast. I yelled and jumped back in pain, and Reptar cackled—actually cackled—before darting down the hall to the kitchen. I rubbed my breast, which was tender enough at the best of times, and Grace busied herself with her plethora of packaging.

'Sorry 'bout that,' she said. 'Jimi's hyper today. Sitting in the car for so long drives him up the wall—'

I heard a crash from the kitchen, and slipped into damage control mode.

'You should have called,' I said, heading for the kitchen. 'Let me know you were coming. I would have—ah—boiled a bagel.' A total lie. Actually, I would have run around like crazy moving breakables up high. A visit from Reptar was a seek-and-destroy mission.

'Well, it was a kind of spur-of-the moment thing.' Grace struggled down the hall with all the bags. Yeah, sure *looked* impromptu. 'When I heard, I just had to come and see you. It's excellent! How far along are you?'

'Eighteen weeks.'

'Eighteen?' she shrieked. 'That's great!'

We arrived at the kitchen. Reptar was at the fridge digging into the Nuttalex container. Grace dropped her bags, went across and extracted his fingers.

'You'll love giving birth,' she said, wiping Reptar's fingers with a tea towel. A *tea towel!* 'It'll change your life. You'll suddenly understand the power of your being.'

I stared into the contaminated Nuttalex. The *power* of my *being?*

'When Jimi was born—well, I was sure glad that Michael was there. It really put him in his place, to see the power of woman like that.' She gave me a god-awful, *we're better than them* wink and added, 'You should have told me!'

Yes, logically, seeing Grace was the only one of our crowd who'd had a baby. I should have gone straight to her for advice and support. I'd told everyone else. Zac, my flatmates, people at work, friends, family, the guy at the milkbar—even complete strangers on the bus. I told every single person I came into contact with.

Except Grace. I'd been avoiding her like rubella.

Because Grace was the Mother of Reptar, without doubt the nastiest piece of three-year-old work I'd ever seen. Some might say that a three-year-old can't be mean, but they haven't seen Reptar in action. He'd stare you in the eye and break your favourite cup, just because he knew you liked it. He'd pull down his pants and shit on your floor, when he *knew* a toilet or potty was available. He'd destroy every room in your house.

He should have carried a public health warning.

And now the creator of this was giving *me* advice.

'You have to give a lot of thought to the delivery. Whatever you do, don't let them give you an epidural—or any drugs for that matter. You don't want the baby's first experience of the world to be on a mind-altering substance.'

Reptar was running his sticky-honey-rice-cake hands through Grace's hair, chanting, 'Mum Mum Mum' in a demented, grating tone.

'In fact,' she continued, 'you should go for a home birth.'

'Well,' I said, 'I thought I'd try the hospital, seeing it's just down the road.'

Grace shook her head, like I was a traitor to the cause. *Her* cause. 'Well, take it from me, I wish I'd done it at home. I mean, they were nice at the hospital, and we had the birthing suite and everything, but next time I'm definitely doing it at home. Preferably in the kitchen, 'cos it's the hive of feminine activity.'

I suppressed a laugh. 'Not in my house.'

'Oh, you could get it organised.' She looked about the small, narrow kitchen as Reptar slid down off her hip. 'Well—maybe you ought to try the lounge room.'

'I think I'll stick with the hospital for now.' I made it sound like I was still considering her idea, but my mind was already made up. I wanted doctors and nurses and *facilities*, but it seemed admitting so would set me up as her inferior. And I didn't even want to be in competition. So I tried to distract her with a story from my last visit to the clinic.

'This doctor came in to give me the results of my Hep and HIV tests, and he looked really, really serious, and I thought, Shit, I've got AIDS! Then he said, "Anna Malcolm?" And I said, "No, Kelly Hedges", and he gave me this really big grin and said, "Oh, there's been a mix-up". So I had to go back to reception. And then I realised—someone else was about to be told she'd tested positive. And I'd been spared. And when I got back to the waiting room, there were all these women sitting around, and I knew one of them was probably Anna Malcolm, and I just thought—well, it could be me.'

Grace stared at me, dumbfounded.

'Full on,' I said, stating the bleeding obvious, 'don't you think?'

'Yeah.'

The story shut her up for a while. We sat down at the tiny kitchen table and cupped our hands around coffee mugs. Grace was full of thought. I was keeping an eye on the clock so I didn't miss *Days of Our Lives*.

'You'll be giving up work,' she said suddenly. 'I suppose.'

'Well—not for a while. I'm only doing three days a week and—it's manageable.'

'Oh, you should. You need the relaxation. From three months onwards, I just slept all day and lolled around the house. Mike brought me all my meals, and I just concentrated on the baby and summoning all my feminine energies.'

How could I tell Grace that I didn't *want* to be a fat lolling couch potato? I didn't *need* to summon my feminine energies. I was not merely The Expectant Mother, a walking biological inevitable. My life was *not* sewn up so neatly.

'Oh, when I first found out I was pregnant,' she continued, eyes glazed, oblivious to my indifference and the fact that Reptar was now throwing vegetables onto the floor, 'it was like—phew!' She threw out her hands in a dramatic show of relief. 'It was like the answer. After all those years of—*doing* all those *things*—like working, hassling for money, going out, having to be—I don't know —*someone*—I realised suddenly I didn't have to do it any more. I didn't have to be out there. It was like I'd been waiting for it all my life.'

It was clear now. *Reptar was her excuse to opt out.*

'Now it's great. Especially when Michael's away at work. I get the space and the peace just to—*be*.'

Reptar was her excuse and he was a total brat.

'The other day, for example, I just wept all day. I just walked around the house with, like—*tears* streaming down my face—it was like all my emotions just—exploded!' She did the dramatic arm gesture thing again. 'And afterwards I felt so—cleansed.'

Reptar was her excuse and that's WHY he was a brat.

I learned a lot from Grace on that first visit.

The pregnancy was conducted in much the same manner as the life Zac and I had carved out for ourselves. Easygoing, she'll be right. We registered for childbirth classes at the hospital, but unfortunately they were held at the same time each week as *The X-Files*. We looked at it this way: this baby was going to be born, no matter what. We knew the aims of the reproductive system. We didn't, however, know the aims of the TV network, or those Pay TV types, and we might not get to see repeats. It was a question of priorities.

Anyway, *Grace* recommended those classes.

Zac and I were doing it *our* way. We didn't paint or carpet or buy furniture or clothes. We set up a bassinet in the corner of our bedroom with some elementary bedding. The rest we'd get as needed. I grew fat with Leila, and she came with us to parties and films and harbour cruises. She showed an affinity for trip hop, kicking like crazy whenever we played Cypress Hill. She got off on the bass, even in the womb.

Of course, *Grace* didn't approve of Cypress Hill, or most of the music I played. On her next visit, when I was six months gone, she gave me music instruction.

'You can't listen to certain music when you're pregnant. It hits you in the solar plexus—it goes straight to the baby. Take Industrial music, for example. It's really dangerous. You don't know what kind of subliminals those people are putting in. It could scar the baby for life.'

Typical Grace. She doesn't care for Throbbing

227

Gristle, so it turns into a crucial baby health issue.

'You have to think about these things, Kelly.'

Meanwhile, Reptar had found Leila's bassinet and was throwing the half-dozen fluffy toys we'd lined it with across the room. Grace smiled, either oblivious to the mess he was making or confident that someone else would clean it up. Reptar, his face set in anger, yanked the head off a purple giraffe then tore down a photo of Harvey Keitel that was by the door.

'Jimi!' I said, more in horror than chastisement. Grace looked at me like I'd whacked him one.

'He's a bit riled up,' she told me, picking him up, trying to contain his wriggling, wrestling form. 'Michael got him all excited before he went to work today, and then he just left—typical! He walks out the door, and I have to deal with the fallout.'

No, I thought to myself as I scooped poor torn Harvey up off the floor. Everyone *else* deals with it too. Because Grace was an active supporter of the children-as-communal-property theory, and she was forever foisting Reptar onto unsuspecting, unwilling babysitters.

It's not that Reptar was *so* bad.

Not *all* the time, anyway.

There were moments, usually when Grace and Michael weren't about, when he'd calm down and you'd see a really sweet, clever, creative three-year-old behind those darting brown eyes. And for a little while you'd feel warm and gooey towards him, and think, aw, he's not so bad. Then he'd pull all the tape out of a cassette, or piss on your bed (from across the room, laughing, congratulating himself on his accuracy), or throw all the fridge magnets on the floor for no other reason than *they were there*.

Oh, God. What if I gave birth to a Reptar?

At 34 weeks, the people where I worked began to get nervous. Every day, I received smiles of surprise when I walked in the office door, like *Wow, Kelly held out another night*. They winced when I negotiated the spiral staircase, and they brought me peaches and little treats. My sister gave me a suitcase of baby clothes, and Zac and I ooohed and aaahed for her benefit as we extracted miniature T-shirts and cutesy cardigans, but as soon as she left, we zipped it up and stored it under the bed. It didn't seem right to be rifling through Leila's things when she wasn't around.

It was superstition, I suppose. I kept thinking about Anna Malcolm, and how very wrong things can go.

At 36 weeks, Grace visited and was shocked that we hadn't prepared.

'Once the baby's here,' she told me, all but waving her finger, 'you won't have the time to get things ready. Resting and breastfeeding, that's all you'll be doing.'

Zac and I gave it some serious thought. Much as I hated to admit it, Grace was right. There *were* certain things that babies really need. We braved the Baby Goods section at the local hypermart, but it was useless. Towel nappies and safety fasteners were the only real essentials. Everything else was just—well, secondary. *Daddy's Little Angel* bibs—yuck. Fifteen-dollar booties—disgusting. The commodities cheapened the event. We bought a new vacuum cleaner instead.

At 38 weeks, Zac thought it would be a good idea if we went to Grace and Michael's for the weekend. I tried to protest with stories of Reptar's wanton destruction—not to mention the bodily fluids thing—but Zac hadn't seen Reptar at his worst. He told me, 'Oh, he's just an energetic nipper. You shoulda seen my brother Toby when he was that age. His room was like a padded cell. The doctor recommended lithium, but my folks didn't want to go with that, 'cos it stunts the growth.'

I'd never met anyone from Zac's family. They emigrated back to England a couple of years ago, all of them: parents, siblings, aunts and uncles, grandparents. Zac was the only one to stay. He told me he didn't really miss them, but I knew with Leila so close, he must crave some familiarity. I guess that's why he had this visit-a-family-in-action bug in his head.

'And so what happened?' I asked him. 'With Toby?'

Zac smiled. 'Well, the folks thought they'd just go with it and see what happened.'

'And?'

'He's eighteen now. And he's still a mad bastard.'

'So what's the moral of the story? Once a Reptar, always a Reptar?'

Zac laughed. 'No. No moral. I just think one weekend observing family life might set your mind to rest.'

Put me off motherhood forever, more like it.

Grace, Michael and Reptar lived in a leafy suburb. Clear footpaths, nature strips, oxygen in the air. The house was an enormous deco affair with lawns and trees—lots of space for Reptar to run wild. *Crush, kill, destroy . . .*

But he didn't. That's the first thing I noticed.

He just sat playing with Lego while the war raged around him.

Grace and Michael were always at each other. To be precise, Grace was always on at Michael, and he was always completely indifferent, infuriating her further. They argued about everything, and they didn't seem to mind if we overheard, let alone Reptar.

The dinner was horrific. The pilaf burnt, the rice didn't absorb and Grace hit the roof.

'It's your fault!' she yelled at Michael. 'You opened the lid!'

'Only for two seconds,' Michael yelled back.

'How many times have I told you—'

'You had the heat up too high.'

'Bullshit!'

'Pilafs have to simmer—'

'Oh, what would you know?'

'I can cook pilafs fine.'

'Yeah, right!'

'I'll show you.' He started rummaging.

'What are you doing?'

'Making a pilaf.'

'You can't do that!'

'I can and I will!'

The three of us were still at the table. Zac and Reptar and I. We looked at each other without expression and then Reptar climbed down off his chair, walked across the room and sat down with his Lego. Grace and Michael shouted and slammed doors, and my heart went out to Reptar. I wanted to take back every mean thought I'd ever had about him. Actually I wanted to take him with us when we left, which was in the taxi, 10 minutes later. All the way home I thought about him, staring into his Lego bucket.

'See?' Zac said. 'The kid's not so bad, is he?'

Reptar was the least of my worries.

What if I gave birth to a *Grace*?

Leila arrived, healthy and beautiful, and on her second day, Grace and Reptar came visiting. Zac was across the road at the other hospital, visiting a friend who'd broken his leg. Grace's first words to me—her very first words—were, 'You'll realise now what a pain men can be. I wish Michael would have an affair with someone and leave.'

I stared at her, the all-singing, all-lecturing expert-at-everything, and realised an awful truth: I was going to have to get rid of her. The stress, the way she and Michael talked when Reptar was around . . . it was too upsetting. For the past two weeks since the dinner at their home, I'd been full of pity for poor Reptar. He was assuming angel status.

Or so I thought.

Till I caught a glimpse of his eyes as he grabbed Leila's empty baby trolley and sent it flying across the ward. The sister was just coming in with the drug trolley, and when she caught sight of the baby-mover coming towards her, she did a double-take. Thinking there was an infant inside, she jumped back, and the drug trolley crashed into the wall and toppled over. Pills and containers went everywhere. A couple of seedy-looking guys who were visiting a woman in the opposite bed looked like all their Christmases had come at once.

'Jimi,' Grace said, 'don't do that. It could be dangerous.'

And he had that crazed glint in his eye, the same as when he was about to stamp yoghurt into the carpet. He opened his mouth and started screaming at the top of his lungs. Grace rushed to quieten him, but it was too late. All over the ward, babies were crying and mothers were disgruntled. Grace patted his back and tried to console him, as if he was beside himself, but Reptar knew *exactly* what he was doing. He stared at me cold-eyed as he wailed. He *knew* that I saw through him, but he kept on yelling.

'Grace,' I told her, above the noise, 'I think you'd better go.'

A couple of nurses standing in the doorway backed up my suggestion.

'Oh, OK,' Grace said. 'Now, make sure you take it easy, and I'll come around next week and stay for a few days to give you a hand.'

'No, no,' I said, 'you don't have to do that.'

'It's all right,' she said, trying to get Reptar into his stroller. 'It's my pleasure.'

'No, Grace, *really*!' I tried to find the right words. 'I just want to—' I struggled. Corny, make it *corny*. 'Well, I feel it's important for me to *bond* with Leila. I think we need some quality time on our own.'

Grace nodded and said, 'You're right.' Reptar was slapping her in the face. As she clipped the restraint, Reptar went completely berserk. He grabbed my bedsheets and started tugging them off. Grace worked him loose and pushed him to the door, where the sister was still picking up pills and packets from the floor. 'I'll give you a call in a week, then.'

I nodded and waved. Grace nodded and waved. While she wasn't watching, Reptar caught hold of a passing woman's catheter hose and pulled it out. The noise was horrendous. Leila slept right through.

It took six months to get the message through to Grace. Each visit was a trauma. Once she came by and told us they were all recovering from a bad stomach bug. Bent over a bucket for 48 hours, she reckoned. The next morning, of course, Zac and I woke up puking. We were sick for days. Leila was fine.

The next visit, I left Leila in the bouncinette for 30 seconds, and when I got back, Reptar was pissing on her. Actually *pissing*.

Grace laughed. She thought it was funny.

The next visit was the final straw. She brought Reptar and the Lego and bags of food and clothes, and it showed all the signs of being a long visit. She told me she'd had a hellish week, because Reptar had been sick with measles.

Measles!

And that's when I learned my first real lesson of motherhood. Aside from the ache that breastfeeding can cause, and the other physical ailments, and the exhaustion and strange dreams . . .

Selfishness. That's what Grace taught me. I stood there watching her and Reptar coughing all over Leila and thought, I'm busting a gut to make it as perfect as possible

235

for her, then I let these people come and spread their germs on her. Why? Because I'm too polite to say what I really think.

I wondered what Anna Malcolm would do. I wondered about her often.

I gave way to self-interest. I took Grace into the kitchen and in a quiet voice—so Reptar wouldn't hear (see, I *was* being considerate)—asked her, 'Can you please take your things and get out of here?'

And she gave me this stare. It was awful. Like, 'Don't you want to join our club?' Like *she* felt sorry for *me*! I helped her carry everything out, dumped it on the porch then slammed the front door. Just so there was no doubt. So she wouldn't come back next week when she had the flu or something else to pass on. I watched them load up the car through the window, and I felt a bit sorry for Reptar. Grace was telling him something. He was kicking the car door. For a three-year-old, he could sure put a good dent in.

This story has a happy ending. Grace and Michael finally split up, and Reptar spends time with both. His destructive behaviour stopped as soon as his parents separated. He still spends a lot of time staring at his Lego, but these days he's constructing. We don't see him very often, due to the fact that Grace is still mad at me for throwing her out of the house that time, but Michael brings him around occasionally, and Leila thinks he's wonderful. He takes delight in making her laugh. Thankfully, he doesn't piss on the bed to do it.

SALLY MCINERNEY
Field Notes on
Sleeping and Waking

I think of childhood now as an unmapped island into whose centre parents are plunged at the moment of their child's birth; we then have to make our way in slow stages from the island's primaeval central swamps through jungle, forest and grasslands to its shores, from which the distant adult world can be seen across shining water: the journey takes at least five years and must be made with the help of the native guides (who were, in my case, twin baby boys).

When my first three children were born (all within the space of 37 months) I had made only sporadic notes about curious and touching things, landmarks and watersheds. I now knew that, without keeping faithful field notes, I would remember very little of the daily detail of life as it was consumed by childhood again: doubly consumed, because this, 11 years later, was life with twins. And so I made notes and took photographs in an effort to find out where my days had gone.

Record-keeping also helped to validate my feeling that I inhabited a foreign, invisible world which nobody would recognise unless they were living in it too. I became an inadvertent amateur anthropologist, trying to interpret the strangeness of the island world into which I had fallen, and perhaps make some discoveries. The ways of thinking are different there. In the island's steamy swamps and jungles, for instance, sleeping at night is neither a natural law nor a social custom.

I kept, or tried to keep, accurate notes on the twins' sleeping and waking patterns, out of incredulity at what night had become for me: a worker's endless shift with no time off. Day and night were no longer divided; there was no access to the dark tunnel of dreams. The notes on sleep were made in the field under rigorous conditions, often being scribbled on stray scraps of paper in the deepest hours of the night as I staggered to and fro between my own bed and the babies' cots while the air shook with wailing. Some were scrawled on the inside covers of bedside novels and childcare books, where I still come across them occasionally as cryptic evidence of the other life I used to lead.

Sometimes, too tired to make notes, I would try to remember the number of times the babies woke and roused me, but had always forgotten the figures by morning. One terrible night the tally-sheet had reached 16 entries, but after that I had not (although still waking and getting out of bed) had energy enough to register a scrawl, a mark or a scratch of pencil on paper. I thought of acquiring an abacus: it might have been easier to move a bead along a wire. A scrap of paper, undated, crinkled and furred from the washing-machine, shows some of the incoherence that afflicted me:

12-1.45
2.45-3.05 I think
4.00-L feed
5.15-M feed
7.15-L feed
8.00-M feed

(So that night I had one hour's sleep, theoretically, between 1.45 am and 2.45 am; then nearly another hour between three am and four am; then three-quarters of an hour from 4.30 am; then an hour-and-a-half from 5.45 am. Not bad! What happened up till midnight I did not record, in this case; presumably the babies were fed and asleep by about eight or nine pm.)

I often used two columns in my note-keeping, one for each child, and tried to register the time as well:

Aged one month—

L	M
2.25 am to 2.45	2.55 am (*I woke him for a feed too: thought that would be the practical, wise thing to do*) 3.15 am then he had wind for a long time
7 am	7 am

Next day—

L	M
—	*midnight* 2.30 am
2.45 am (*woke him for a feed: wise?*)
—	5 am
6 am	6 am to 8 am (*he had wind, or colic, or something*)

A few days later—

I fed them both from 6 pm to 7 pm, then they were very colicky, both screaming together for an hour or more. So

from about 7 pm to 9 pm, I tried to settle them to sleep.
Midnight: both woke and were fed.
3.30 am: both woke and were fed
7 am to 8 am: as above
. . . A rough night.

Next evening—

Both were fed at about 8 pm and eventually went to sleep.
12.30 am to 1.30 am: both woke, fed, one after the other.
But for a while neither could settle, so in the end it was
12.30 am to 3 am, and then 4 am to 5 am.
The ensuing day was very hot, the height of summer.
Somehow we reeled through it.

Once the babies began to cry at night, they would not
stop. It was not a matter of waiting for a little crying to
diminish: left to develop it would become a desperate
crescendo, impossible to ignore. Occasionally an observer
(father, mother, teenage sister or brother) would be in
the room when the crying began: we would see how the
peacefully sleeping child began to twist and wriggle, his
face contorting, the cry breaking from his lips, his eyes
still fastened shut in sleep: it was so obviously not casual
or wilful. The trouble (colic, dreams or demons) seized

him, shook him into waking with a cry for comfort. And the comfort, for a very long time, meant breastfeeding: as if the depths of the babies' unconscious, combined with the depths of their troubled digestive systems, created a need not simply for human contact but for a kind of actual fusion with human life, a reassurance that could only be obtained by taking part of the mother's body into their own. Having been hauled out of the dark bucket of nightmares and existential frights, they were reattaching themselves to life by latching onto the breast. It was the thing both babies seemed most fervently to want, and an unfailing means of bringing about peace for all parties— until the next time.

That's how it seemed; and I complied, for breastfeeding was reassuring to me as well, as a way of communicating with such embryonic, enigmatic souls. I didn't want to risk destroying, by letting them scream on, the inherent hope they presumably had of the world. (For surely when a very young, helpless creature feels pain—hunger, colic, cold—then the pain brings fear of death, which is a very good reason for crying.) Bottles of milk, water, dummies, walking, talking, singing, rocking—none of these traditional soothing devices worked. As a substitute for breasts, bottles were of no interest to them: we tried, but in the early, most crucial stages they would simply reject the rubber teat and scream for the human one. I kept expecting them to lose interest in breastfeeding and to wean themselves, as the others had done, but the natural rivalry of twins (or so I concluded, after many months) meant that neither would be first to give up seizing and reclaiming his share of the mother-territory. And so it went on.

Besides, I could never sleep to the sound of crying.

Aged four-and-a-half months—

> 6 pm: *they fed, then went to bed . . . quite happily, then slept till 5.50 am!! Their best record so far.*

At the time we thought that this was the breakthrough; the fogs of exhaustion might be about to clear. But about two weeks later the babies began waking up at night, often three times each. Teeth, wind, hunger, dreams? Or a combination of these, with perhaps another factor which I noted at the time: . . . *they* like *waking up at night?* But then, hovering silently above their cots, we would observe again the disturbed and painful waking described above: it was clear that their sleep was being troubled and broken, their waking was not wilful, and they definitely needed comforting when it happened.

After five months, we began feeding them 'solids', mainly because they had begun to open their mouths like young birds whenever they watched adults eating. A month later—although by this stage they were wolfing down mashed vegetables, stewed fruit, cereal, and graciously accepting a bottle of formula milk if I were out somewhere— they were still both breastfed, and made their wishes for this very clear by crying and shoving the proffered bottle or 'solids' aside, making a beeline for me, grabbing and climbing onto me, putting their hands down my shirt and desperately twisting to seize a nipple, and so on.

At eight-and-a-half months—

Three meals a day—yep—and at night . . . chaos!
Last night: both woke and wailed . . . before midnight.
Then at 1 am Max woke; woke again at 3 am; woke Leo;
I fed them both; then both woke again at 6 am and romped
around happily in their cots . . . When they wake, it's not
hunger particularly but seems to be wind, or teeth, or
both . . .

This was not a case of petulant infants imperiously summoning their parent-slaves. There was true urgency in their cries; and so we always attended to them, until they were old enough to take note of our reasonable voices calling from the next room: 'Please let us sleep a little bit longer . . . We'll be there soon'; but by this time, anyway, they were walking and almost talking and no

longer emitting those unearthly desperate cries that
overturn adults' hearts. And by this time a father's
comforting voice and arms were just as effective as a
mother's, if not more so.

At 12 months—

> *We are very tired, we think, tireder than we know . . .*
> *11 pm: both woke briefly . . .*
> *12-1 am: both woke . . .*
> *3-3.30 am: L fed and into cot*
> *4.45-5 am: M fed and into cot.*
> *5.30-5.40: M bumped head on cot and woke*
> *5.50: L woke crying*
> *5.55: M woke crying . . . walked him for 10 mins and he*
> *went back to sleep*

After one year, we decided to try the desperate remedies
calmly recommended in certain baby-care books, and
'train' the babies out of their frequent night wakings. We
thought that doses of an infant-tailored sedative on going
to bed might break their habit of waking throughout the
night; this was to be combined with 'controlled crying'
when they were first put to bed (where the adults respond
to the initial wails, but with ever-increasing intervals

between responses, so that the infants eventually give up issuing the parent-summons, knowing that they are close at hand though slow to arrive). The controlled crying method helped us to get them to sleep in the first place, but they kept waking up thereafter.

At 13 months—

Well, despite the doses of Phenergan we gave them [at bedtime] *recently they both continue to wake—on a very good night perhaps only three times (this is very rare) and usually a) a couple of times each after they go to bed and before we do, and then b) between two and four times each after that and before dawn . . . They almost always have one or two sleeps during the day—a three-hour stint is not extraordinary.*

[These sleeps, of course, did not always occur simultaneously.]

We soon gave up the practice of sedating them, having tried it on perhaps six occasions to little effect. Inevitably, they still woke up several times during the night and cried. We felt, anyway, a deep unease at chemically manipulating them—no matter how harmless it might really be, and how broken the nights. It seemed the ultimate act of bullying: they so small, trusting and innocent, we with our huge stature slipping sleeping-draughts down their throats when they opened their bird-like mouths. Things would get better, we knew.

At 15 months—

	M	L
[time not recorded]	1	—
[time not recorded]	—	1
12.30 am	1	1
[time not recorded]	—	1
3.30 am	1	1
4.30 am	1	1
5.30 am	1	1

(*total – 11 wakings*)

At 16 months—

Some rough nights, some smooth ones where one baby (either one) sleeps all night—ie: 7 pm to 6 am. This has happened about five times since they were born. I'm still breastfeeding them because I can't see how not to. During the day they'll climb onto my lap and swivel their legs around (L has the left side, M the right). Will this one-sidedness affect each of them permanently? . . . And what about the [developing] *hemispheres of their brains?* [I could find no one to answer these questions.]

Was it my fault? Should I have forcibly weaned them? Was I a misguided sucker? I thought about all this, knowing that when infants give their mothers trouble, the mothers generally take the blame for being bad managers. But there was no escaping the facts: the infants woke at night because they could not help doing so; and their desire to keep on being breastfed was unequivocal.

When they were nearly 18 months old, we took them, because we had to, across the Pacific on a plane. They slept, but never simultaneously, so we were awake and watchful for 16 hours. In London, dazed by jetlag and lack of sleep, I saw only one child amongst us and screamed, 'Oh, God, where's the other one?' Panic-stricken and furious, I could not understand why nobody else in the party seemed alarmed. They looked back bemusedly at me and finally somebody said, 'He's in your arms'. In the decrepit London hotel, they proved forever that jetlag is not a psychological condition by waking every morning at two, and scampering across the floors until the management rang to say that all the people below were complaining. Outside it was pitch black and very cold, but the infants were ready to greet the day. At two in the afternoon they would fall into a leaden slumber, and I would wander out alone, dazed and dishevelled, to gaze through unfocused eyes at the fabled sights of London.

Back on home ground, I made a progress report at 18 months—

6.30 am: Max is up (since 6 am) and Leo is calling out from his cot and M is occasionally answering him. At night they go cheerfully into their cots—usually—instead of screaming brokenheartedly as they used to. We stay and sing to them or pat them, drifting in and out of the room still singing so we are heard though not seen. Sometimes they even indicate that they want to lie down, by leaning and steering us adults towards the cots when we are carrying them.

However, by about midnight they begin to wake: they then stand up in their cots and cry till rescue comes. If it's me who comes [and for the six weeks when their father was away working in Hungary, for instance, it was always me], *then nothing but a 'feed' will persuade them to go back to sleep. Sometimes one wakes the other and then, if I am alone, I feed them both even if it's 3 am. Sometimes they wake separately, perhaps three times each.*

The first time both children slept all night—well, till five am—with neither one waking, was just two months before their second birthday. We were asleep at the time, naturally, so this momentous event escaped us like an eclipse of the moon obscured by cloud.

At 25 months—

Both wake about 5 or 6 am . . . and often go back to sleep.
They sleep for 2-3 hours from about 1 pm.
They go to sleep again about 7.30, 8 or even 9 pm.
Both often wake at 2 or 3 am, have a drink of water and go back to sleep (unless woken by mosquitoes, teeth or dreams).

For at least two years I was crazed and dazed from lack of sleep; I lost the art of dreaming and even of sleeping, for my ears were always tuned to the sounds of little children and so I could never feel alone enough to sink into true sleep. (Other people's babies, and indeed my own three older children, when they were babies—as far as I could remember—were famously untroubled sleepers. Other babies, including my own first three, weaned themselves efficiently before 12 months were up.)

I would welcome the first bars of daylight because the endless work seemed easier then; light made my life seem almost normal, and sometimes I would take an early-waking baby to the car (bundling him up hastily before his brother woke too), and then, as pale new sunlight began to wash the tops of buildings and when the traffic lights were almost always green, we would drive through the centre of the city, seeing strange men surreptitiously open the doors of vans to let giant factory guard dogs, coming off night duty, bound through grassy parks where office workers would later gather to seize a slice of midday sun; and the shining snail-tracks of street-washing council trucks; and the men and women carrying buckets and rags, who unlock and clean huge deserted buildings for people they never meet. I felt a kinship with this secret army of shiftworkers, though I was one with no appointed knock-off time. It was comforting to see other people to whose labour the enormous world of daylight normality was almost oblivious; though the night workers in turn were oblivious to me—only a passing driver with a baby cocooned in the back seat.

These early-morning runs through the heart of the city, when it was at its most tender, quiet and renewed, consoled me as if—though my life excluded me from normal life—I had slipped into the centre of that other world through an inconspicuous side path. And one morning my little passenger seemed so happy, so entertained, that I ventured even further into the lost territory and took him (in his

253

stripy one-piece pyjamas like a jumping bean) to an Italian coffee shop in a rough back street, an early-opener for hard-working men who gave him kind and quizzical looks as they leaned over their coffees, stirring in lots of sugar. He and I were alien creatures, very happy to have arrived on Earth for a while.

By the age of three the children usually slept all night, sometimes waking long after sunrise. With each other for company, they went to bed quite cheerfully, around eight pm, sitting up in bed and 'reading'. At last there was an established domestic ceremony known as bedtime, in between daytime and night-time (the long arms of the clock were already catching hold of their lives). We generally read, or told, stories to them at bedtime. A sense of sanity slowly began to return.

And so the sleep saga came quietly to a close, and I re-entered the world of the normal living; but for a long time afterwards, amongst crowds of people in brightly lit rooms, people who had no babies in their current lives, or no sympathetic imagination, I often felt that I had emerged from a shadowy place that had claimed or captured several years of my life, so that my world-experience was different to theirs; and the indefinable stamp was on me, of someone who had 'been away', in a foreign country, or a foreign state of mind.

(Adapted from *Leaving the Island*, forthcoming.)

KERRY CUE
War of the Words!

I t happened on a dull winter day in Melbourne as depression gripped a lifeless suburbia like a ground-hugging fog. I stood at the school gate, an extra raincoat in hand, and waited. The bell rang. Suddenly an explosion of youthful vitality poured out of the school building, filling the grey streetscape with exuberance and laughter.

I saw my child. Torn T-shirt. Windcheater lost. Most likely. Again. Mud-spattered pants. Shoelaces undone. Dragging the school bag through every available puddle. But there was no exuberant glow on this scrunched-up face. I could read the signs. I could see the dark clouds of anger brewing.

The school bag was thrown at me.

'What's the matter?' I asked.

255

'Everybody in my whole grade can read more better than me.'

And I felt the pain that mothers feel when their child is suffering in any way. I felt the pull of the umbilical cord as it tightened its grip on my heart.

But to tell this story as it should be told, I must back up several years to the time when this child started school. Anxiety—my anxiety—about this deadly-serious business of learning to read began in small ways. Bulletins would arrive from school expressing—in almost hyperventilating tones—the absolute urgency associated with getting children to read. Thirty minutes a day. Children should read 30 minutes a day. I was lucky if my child accumulated 30 seconds reading time over a full week.

Parent-teacher meetings were held. Readers discussed. Children were issued with a cover for readers containing, in the back, a record of titles and dates. My child lost the cover.

Parental help was sought to hear reading. I volunteered. I went to the school and heard other people's children read, while my child sat under the table prising dried chewing gum off the chipboard. I was knee deep in bright-eyed Emmas and Kates who had read 34 *I-Can-Read* books each—probably before breakfast— and were expressing a keen interest in moving on to chapter books. Meanwhile my child showed a consistent lack of interest in even looking at the pictures in picture books. Except the book about sharks. My child particularly liked the picture of the shark gnawing off someone's leg.

More bulletins arrived home citing the strong correlation between literacy levels and future success. I was becoming quite anxious about my child, who seemed to show great interest in collecting rubber bands, pencil shavings, odd-shaped stones and broken sticks, and no interest whatsoever in things like future success.

Parents were reminded that they were now expected to take an active role in their children's education. Providing children with a sound genetic make-up was no longer enough. It was now up to parents to improve their children's educational lot as well.

Parents must be there academically. Children, after all, only spend six hours a day at school. What of the other 18 hours? The answer was obvious. If parents want their children to get ahead, parents must teach.

The time had come, I felt, to kick my child's learning curve up the vertical axis. I would become involved. Unfortunately, helping my child learn to read was a far more complex matter than I had originally imagined.

The first night of my excessive-parental enthusiasm saw me facing a significant problem. Finding the reader. 'Where IS your reader?' 'In my bag,' was the reply. I searched. I found six stumps of crayons, half a squashed vegemite sandwich, an apple with one bite out of it, someone else's windcheater, 24 rubber bands, eight torn and scrunched-up work sheets—five on tables (unfinished), three on geometric shapes (unfinished) and one on Italy (blank)—and no reader.

I tipped everything out of the bag. I found the reader stuck to the bottom of the bag with a layer of last week's yoghurt. After a quick sponge down of the reader and a fumigation of the school bag, we were ready to begin.

Let me rephrase that. I was ready to begin. My child was outside in the front garden running and skidding along on the knees through various patches of mud. 'Come in and do some reading,' I called.

'What for?' my child called back. I clenched my teeth. 'What for?' My brain was a swirling brew of emotion. 'What for?' I thought. 'So that you can grow up to be a neurosurgeon, that's what for.' But I had to couch this expectation in kid terms. 'Because it's fun,' I said, looking as jolly as death on a day out.

'Look what I can do,' my child called. I looked. My child hung upside down from the Roman rings in the tree. Swinging on the Tarzan rope, my child got tangled in the rope ladder. I had to unknot the rope from those grubby legs.

'Now come inside,' I urged with a shallow enthusiasm. We went. 'I've found your reader,' I said to my child, who was on the floor with the Lego. 'Let's read.' My child ignored me. 'Let's read,' I hissed.

'Wha?'

'I have found your reader.'

'Ugh.' My child's attention returned to the Lego.

'Catch,' I called, knowing there would be a response. My child turned and caught the book. The child is quick, and grasped what was going on. The book was thrown back to me. 'No. You read it,' I said, throwing the book in the child's direction. 'You,' came the insistent reply, as it was thrown back again.

After four throws I had to ask myself, What are you doing? Trying to teach your child to read by the Frisbee Method? It didn't seem to be working. But the day was young. I would trap the child in bed.

I sat beside the bed. 'Look at this,' I said. '*Frog and Toad are Friends.*'

'Yuk!' was the reply.

'Don't you like frog and toad?'

'No. I don't like the book.'

'Well, why did you pick it?'

'I didn't pick it. She (the teacher, esteemed Mrs X) made me take it.'

'Oh. I see. I tell you what. You pick a book. And tomorrow night we'll read it.'

Next day at school, at the gate, I opened the school bag. Bingo. My child had picked a book. *Mrs Wishy Washy*. I remember it well. That night I sat beside my child on the bed. 'OK. Let's read *Mrs Wishy Washy*,' I chortled. And my child read it. Word perfectly. Cover to cover. I was stunned. Not so much that my child had read a book, but because my child had read the book without actually looking at it. My child was looking at a

Disney poster on the wall. My child had read the book by ear. My genius child had memorised it.

'Very good,' I said with two-star approval ringing in my voice. 'Tomorrow night, we'll read another book.'

'No,' replied my child. 'I only want to read this one.'

'We'll read another one,' I insisted through gritted teeth.

Next day, at the school gate. Bingo. Another book. Good on vigilant Mrs X. We were cohorts in this literacy conspiracy. That night I sat by my child's bed. I took out the reader. 'Here we go,' I enthused. My child looked at the book. And sighed. My child lolled backwards and plopped onto the pillow. Not to be outdone, I lay down beside my child and held the book in front of the yawning face. My child flopped an arm over the bed, then rolled out of bed onto the floor.

I was not about to be deterred. I do not suffer deterrence easily. I lay on the bed and held the book in front of my child's face on the floor. My child looked up and began to kick the book. Tempers were fraying here. The tension could be cut with a pair of child-safe scissors.

Then it happened. The tantrum. 'I hate it. I hate it. I hate reading. I don't want to do it ever again.'

Unfortunately, that was me. I had snapped.

I'd endured several months and many, many attempts to entice this child to read. This child wasn't about to be enticed. I was forcing the issue. Ve Hav Vays to make you read. There can be no escape. But I wished I hadn't snapped. I may have sent my child's learning curve plunging into the negatives.

I wanted my child to learn to read. Desperately. But through these many months of persistence, I felt uneasy. Unsettling questions kept gnawing at the core of my resolve. Do I really have to do this? Do I have to invade every zone of my offspring's childhood with measuring tapes and yardsticks? Do I have to weigh down, even burst, that free-floating bubble called childhood with my hefty expectations? Why do I feel so guilty about trying to make my child learn to read?

At least, I knew the answer to that last question. I felt guilty loading up my offspring's childhood with burdens of educational responsibility for the simple reason that my own childhood had been free of such burdens.

My parents were interested in my education. I knew that. On Education Day, my mother would put on her hat and coat and visit my primary school. It was the 1950s. And education was a straightforward concept. Health involved simply cutting out pictures of carrots and sticking them in an exercise book. Learning to read involved listening to 35 or more kids in the grade read one line each, one at a time. If you could stomach it. If not, you looked out the window and chewed the end of your pencil.

But once a year, religiously, my mother would visit the school and view the display containing my one page of good work. And every year she would say, 'Very good'. Then she skedaddled on home and kept out of my education for another year. I appreciated her involvement. Later on, I grew to appreciate her lack of involvement more. She was there in my education if I asked for help. But she never arrived uninvited with boxes of worthy books under her arm.

So I felt guilty. I felt guilty because I was storming my child's education armed with great authority and even greater expectations and I didn't like what I was becoming—a card carrying member of the Academic Gestapo. I didn't want to whip my child, metaphorically or otherwise, through those 12 long years of school education.

Besides, I knew deep down why my child wasn't reading. It was a mother's instinct calling to me. It may have been buried beneath many layers of concrete advice but I could still hear the cry. This child is smart. Brilliant at times. This child is also stubborn, determined and relentless. This child doesn't read because this pint-sized dynamo hasn't sat still long enough to focus on the printed word.

So, when some months later that accusing face looked up to me on that cold and bleak winter's day, I held true to my mother instinct. 'Listen kiddo,' I said. 'If you want to learn to read you have to run those eyeballs of yours across some printed words from time to time. It's that simple.'

And I can report that I didn't have to drag, carry or force my child into literacy. The time had come to learn to read. And my child learned.

It was the one clear vision of certainty I've had in motherhood. And I was thankful for it.

CANDIDA BAKER
Just a Little One, Dear

My mother did not live to see my son, her grandson born. When he somewhat belatedly chose to make an appearance into the world, it was on the day before my mother's birthday, and somehow this made it particularly poignant for me.

I'm not quite sure why, because to tell the truth, even if she had been alive she would have been less than useful as a grandmother, as indeed she had become less than useful as a mother. But somehow, when Sam was born, this knowledge did not lessen my sense of loss. I wanted my mother to see my boy-child—I am one of four girls, and my sister has two daughters; I was absolutely convinced that I was carrying a girl, and delighted when I gave birth to a hefty 10-pound boy. I wanted her to have seen me get married to the man I had lived with for 10 years. I wanted her, I suppose, to acknowledge my achievements, and I wanted all this from a mother who had become incapable of emotional connection.

It is a terrible thing to have parental love snatched away, either by divorce or death, or by a breakdown, or, in some sad cases, by inertia or entropy. In my case, it was not so much that it was snatched away, more that it was eroded over time by the canker of my mother's alcoholism.

I am the adult child of an alcoholic.

I remember the first time the phrase hit home. I was 34, already well down my recovery path, or so I thought at the time. Then one night I was sitting at the dining room table, flicking through a magazine, when I chanced across an article about adult children of alcoholics.

'You will recognise yourself as the adult child of an alcoholic,' the article said, 'if you have trouble with:

a) long term commitment
b) decision-making
c) telling the truth
d) understanding priorities
e) saying what you feel
f) anger.'

(Or they were words to this effect, anyway.)

As I sat at the table I began to cry. I cried because despite the steps I had already taken to recover from dysfunctional and chaotic parenting, I was suddenly pierced with the knowledge that this was something from which there was no complete recovery. Just as my mother remained an alcoholic, I would, in some part of me, remain the adult child of an alcoholic. And although my mother was not yet then dead, I cried for her, for the love I had received from her before she succumbed to her dis-ease, and for her wasted life, and I cried with anger because I wanted that love back, and it was not and never would be again, available to me.

Sometimes, in the first year of Sam's life, I would be filled with an unutterable sadness. Perhaps it was postnatal depression, or a form of it anyway. But I was someone who had reached the age of 34 with no close acquaintance with death, other than my maternal grandmother when I was a child. Within the space of two years my mother died, my father's mother died, my uncle died, and my step-mother who had been with my father for nearly 30 years, also died, shortly after Sam was born. Sometimes I would sit with this tiny baby on my lap and for the first time in my life I would question what on earth the point of it all was. I did not feel exactly suicidal but I felt very alone and somehow having a child enhanced those feelings. I felt as if I had never needed a mother more, and that there was no one I could turn to who would understand. I felt angry that I had lost my mother twice, once from drink, once from death. It seemed to me that the burden of her alcoholism had not only been passed to me, but even to my child, who was the child of an adult child of an alcoholic.

This is not to say that my mother became an alcoholic and stopped loving her children, not at all. But her love for us, as with the rest of her life, became warped in fantasy. From the time I was a teenager, it was as if the roles had been reversed—as the adult I would try to coax the child gently towards reality, and she, with increasing cleverness, would resist. When I once tackled her about her loneliness, living in a four-bedroom cottage by herself, with no job, no car and no company, she gently chided me in a letter: 'What with doing my own washing and feeding the birds, I keep very busy.' If the expression had existed at the time, I might well have responded with: 'Mum, hellooo?'

These days I wonder what chance she ever had. Her father was an alcoholic and he was not the first in the family, according to my uncle (who also told me that we even have a de-frocked priest in a cupboard which is a bit too full of skeletons for my liking). My father has always enjoyed a drink, and alcohol was a major part of our family life—when we were children our father gave us diluted red wine to 'nourish' us, and as we grew older drinking was positively encouraged.

It bothers me a bit that Sam's and my mother's birthdays are so close together. Often I've thought, 'What if he has the gene?' These days he's a healthy and lively four-year-old, and it's absurd to imagine that he and she are linked in that way, but I still worry about it. One thing I know is that he won't be given red wine at lunchtime!

I'm not sure why my mother stepped over the line that separates a drinker from an alcoholic. I used to think that the rot set in the day my father had a heart attack and we discovered at the same time that his mistress, who was staying in our house, was pregnant with his child, and that she had been his mistress for the past five years. I used to think that perhaps it began when the fairytale life we lived until I was eight ended as abruptly for her as it did for me, when we moved from a comfortable flat in London's Belgravia to our hitherto weekend cottage in a small Oxfordshire hamlet with no shops. There, in a crowded damp cottage, my mother with four children under the age of eight, two of them twins, with no driving licence and a flourishing career as a dress designer cut off in full swing, fell, I suppose, into a gentlewoman's decline of a particularly English kind. For a long time, after I emigrated to Australia at the age of 22, I had a hidden and horrible belief that it was my departure that caused it, that if I had stayed in England I might have prevented her from becoming an alcoholic.

Alcoholics are, like any addicts, extremely cunning. They are also very good at persuading themselves and those around them that they are not alcoholics. As a teenager I finally managed to persuade our family doctor that Mum might have a problem. I coaxed my mother into the surgery to see him. She came out delighted, and armed with several prescriptions—one for amphetamines because she wanted to lose weight and she was tired, one for Valium to help her stay calm, and one for Mogadon to help her sleep at night. That combined with no lessening of alcoholic intake caused her to become almost zombie-like. She lost weight all right—she was either too manic, too drunk or too stoned to eat. A few years later she did manage, to her credit, to go cold turkey on the pills, showing a latent willpower she could never extend to booze and fags, but at the time what most horrified me was the way she had hoodwinked the doctor. I was roundly told off both by him, and later by my mother, for even suggesting that she had a drink problem when the problem was her difficult (and at the time, rightly or wrongly, I read: *Include you lot in this statement*) life.

It was the first in a long line of hoodwinks which became second nature to her, so that even up until the time she died there were friends of hers who were surprised when the second cause of death on the autopsy was cirrhosis of the liver. The first, and as it happened, by far the kindest, being a fall down her steep cottage stairs early in the morning when she broke her neck.

And this was the mother, now lying on the cold tile floor with her leg twisted up under her, her neck broken and massive bruises on her head, who had loved me so much and so well when I was a child, that if I am in any way a half-decent mother, it is because of her early nurturing.

What I found as Sam grew older was that through my mothering of him I rediscovered my own mother's mothering, and that has become a source of great joy to me. Every time we get the paints out, or make a delicious mess in the kitchen, or play in the park or even settle down to watch a program together, I remember how she was when I was a child, and it is almost as if her voice speaks through me. I like that voice. It's not the same thing as occasionally sounding like one of my parents and thinking, 'Oh God, I sound exactly like my parents!'— it's a nurturing voice that I used to love from her and now love to give to Sam. She would read and then sing to me at night, and I do this with him every night with a great sense of gratitude that we have these rituals in the family.

I still have problems reconciling the two extremes of my mother's life. So, too, do her oldest friends. On my last visit to England one of them said to me, 'The thing about Julia was she was so ambitious. She might not have been the cleverest girl in the school, but she was the most ambitious. She always knew what she wanted'.

What she wanted, and what she had, to a large degree, achieved by the time I was born, was a successful career as a film costume designer. Mine was, apart from the unpredictability of my father's temper, a privileged childhood. An elegant flat, two Siamese cats, a film-star father and all the accompanying treats, like smocked dresses made by the Queen's dressmaker, with, heaven forfend, matching bloomers! Walks in St James Park with the nanny, and the new baby in the pram. A private pre-school where we learned French and ballet, and from which I would dash home to watch *Crackerjack* and kiss John Lennon on the television screen. Weekends were spent in the country, first at other people's cottages, and then at our own, collecting eggs, playing on the farm, learning to ride and messing about by the river. It would be tempting to say it was idyllic, and certainly there was a lot about it that nourished and nurtured me, but it was already a facade. Chaos and unpredictability were never far from the surface, and yet, like many other English children, what I learned was that everything must at least look perfect—if the silver is gleaming then God (English, of course) is in his heaven, and all's right with the world.

However, there are things my mother taught me in my early childhood that have stayed with me right through my life—that it's OK for children to make a big mess in the kitchen; how (I hope!) to be kind and comforting; how important food and a clean (well, clean-ish) house are; and how important rituals are for family well-being.

By the time I was a teenager this was all well and truly gone. It had become impossible for her to hold down a job—each attempt was thwarted by her drinking. There had been the move to the country, a move back to London in an attempt to save the marriage, a return to the country. I moved in with my grandmother in London and would visit at the weekend. A financial pattern was established—I would bring money, my mother would spend it. She would, it seemed to me, extract money out of me by osmosis. By now visits from the bailiff had become regular occurrences; it was hard to keep up with the electricity and the phone as they were cut off so often. Around this time, too, one of my younger sisters was admitted to hospital suffering from malnutrition and kidney failure. Malnutrition!

I would be gilding the lily if I said that I had inherited only good mothering from my mother. How could that be, when her mothering became so erratic, and finally non-existent? For a long time I found that I was not very good at setting boundaries for Sam, or indeed for myself around Sam. I found—still find—that if we go to a shop and I have money, I feel as if I should spend it on him. My mother, increasingly childlike, became a great one for 'treaties', and if her daughters were in any way unpleasant to her, we were made to understand that it could be made up to her with a 'treat'. Often, after I've told Sam off, I'm filled with an overwhelming desire to spoil him to an equal degree. Sometimes I'm shocked to realise that he has manipulated me in exactly the same way she used to—first my mother, now my child! The process of taking control of these situations is sometimes slow and difficult— reversing decades of behaviour, but it's worth it, every painful step.

One day when we were in the process of taking a valuable corner cupboard off the wall to sell to pay the debts, my mother collapsed in tears. The only alternative, I suggested—and she agreed—was for us to go to her wealthy brother, my uncle, and tell him everything, including her drinking problem.

It was as if we had waved a magic wand. He provided credit at the shop for food, he paid the bills, he sent her to her first stint in a drying out home and we all had such high in the sky, apple-pie hopes.

Later my uncle's help proved to be a mixed blessing. People say that alcoholics must hit their own rock bottom before they can make the choice to climb out. My mother's journey through life was now cushioned. With her brother there for the rest of her life, to pay for her visits to Australia, to pay for her 'little holidays', as she called them, at Champneys (non-drying out home of the rich and famous), I suppose we took that chance away from her. I suspect it has been held against me, perhaps I have held it against me too, but I was little more than a child myself and I did my best at the time.

I'm not sure how long it was after my uncle stepped in that I realised there was no hope. Not long, I suspect. The doctors at Champneys had recommended that she visit AA (as if AA was something you could simply pop into from time to time!). When she showed no signs of complying with this suggestion I asked her why she wouldn't go. 'But darling,' she said, 'Oxford! I ask you. I mean, if it was Belgravia I might go, but *Oxford*.' Up until then I had always thought that she wanted to give up drinking as much as we wanted her to, but this, too, was suddenly shown to be a sham. Many years later after one of her other 'little holidays', in a suddenly wicked mood she regaled one of my sisters with tales of how she and the other regular patients had learned how to outwit the doctors and nip into the local pub for a drink!

My mother had always wanted to be wealthy, had always wanted a career and a certain status in life. With the help of my uncle's money, she slipped further and further into her fantasy. She would order the most expensive smoked salmon from the corner store, or ring us up and ask us to 'bring home a pound of fresh lychees from Harrods, darling'—this last in the middle of winter. I think she even persuaded herself that my father's marriage to my step-mother was just a minor aberration in what my mother saw as her continuing relationship with him. Even after 27 years of my father's relationship with my step-mother, my mother would say, 'Of course, she doesn't know how to manage him. You have to know, with your father, how to handle him'. Yes, Mum.

The dichotomies were endless. The woman who had once designed and made all her own clothes wore her sister-in-law's cast offs. The woman who had once insisted that we iron the flannels, underpants, socks and sheets, lived in a house where the iron was covered in spider webs.

Quite frankly, I can't think how she did keep her family, the house and the garden together for so long. No wonder it drove her to drink. It's some years since I tried to keep a completely clean house, I must admit, and to say that standards have dropped since Sam was born would be an understatement. Sometimes I look around our house and find it resembles a bomb-site. The only time the iron sees the light of day is when a visitor comes to stay. Sam is always very curious about it, and insists on playing with the ironing board. *Sometimes the ornaments have not one but several layers of dust on them!* What I have learned is that I simply can't hold down a fulltime job, look after a child, try to find time to do my own writing, and have the world's cleanest house. There is absolutely no point trying.

After my mother's death, after the village funeral and the village wake, after a few days there with my sisters, I had some time on my own in my childhood home. We all reacted to her death in very different ways. I was so angry that I set about trying to eradicate all traces of dirt from the cottage. There was shit on her carpet, in her bed, there were bottles stacked up everywhere. It was the death of a sloven, and I was furious with her. Over the years I had of course seen the gradual decline of the house from the ironing and brass-cleaning frenzy of my childhood, but now on close examination it was so horribly obvious— silverfish, spiders, dirt an inch thick, everything squalid and slimy and disgusting. And yet, just occasionally, something perfect: her neat and tidy drawers full of tools, everything in their right place and a right place for everything, just as when we were children.

One of the things I discovered, or believe I discovered, about Mum after Sam was born was that she, like me, was actually bored by a great deal of the motherhood experience. It was almost as if I could feel her anger and impotence at not being able to get on with her drawing and painting within my own anger at not being able to find time to write. My sister had discovered through her own postnatal depression that Mum had, she felt, suffered badly from postnatal depression after her and her twin's birth. Not really surprising, given the circumstances of my father's already existing affair at the time.

The oddest thing about having an alcoholic parent is that it is commedia dell'arte writ large. It is tragic but it is also comic. Sometimes the comedy strikes you at the time, sometimes afterwards. Is it some strange life-saving mechanism set up so that we don't actually murder or cut off forever from the ones we love? How can you be forever angry at the person who drinks a whole bottle of duty-free Chivas Regal, replaces it with cold tea, and pretends stoutly that she has done nothing to it, and insists, 'There must have been something wrong with it dear'. It's just not possible. It is, of course, remarkably similar to having a child isn't it? The shock, and the inevitable laughter as you discover that your favourite lipstick has been used as body-paint, or that the child has decided to pour two litres of apple juice into the dog's bowl. Why? I suppose the answer is the same for Sam, as for my mother when faced with a bottle: Why not?

These days, in my 40s, I actually hold onto these funny memories. I have many memories of my mother sober, but in many ways to deny the alcoholic memories is to deny who she chose to be. There was the time I took my Australian partner to meet her for the first time and she fell down the stairs (yes, the same stairs) and landed at his feet. There was the time she said she wanted to come and see a preview of a Jack Nicholson and Meryl Streep film with me, and was drunk by the time I had to leave; but I insisted (how ridiculous) that she come anyway, and then refused to help her, so that she had to negotiate her way down the street holding onto the railings. When we arrived at the theatrette, I had forbidden her to ask for a drink, on the pain of death, but as the cheerful PR girl asked if we would like a mineral water, or tea or coffee, my mother smiled sweetly, if lopsidedly, and said, 'How kind of you. I'd love a nice glass of white wine if you have it'. I was furious. My mother turned her innocently owlish eyes on me. 'Just a little one, dear,' she said. As we sat down in the dark I snatched the glass away from her and drank the lot! Which was probably a good thing since when the film started it was *Ironweed*. I sank further and further into a guilty gloom—how could I possibly have brought my mother to this! She, sensing victory, asked for another white wine, and the diabolically true to life—gentlewoman becomes alcoholic, fucks up her life and dies—subject matter was never referred to. All she said was that she thought Meryl Streep wasn't at her best! 'The trouble with Meryl Streep,' she said afterwards, 'is that she's horsy.'

There are the awful memories, too, of course. Rushing to her shopping when she arrived home from the shops (before she was banned from driving forever after causing a fearful collision on the Banbury Road) and pouring the whisky down the sink. Why on earth did we bother? She always found more anyway. Or arriving home from school into a darkened house where the smell of cigarettes and whisky would immediately alert me as to her state that day. Or her crying drunkenly in her chair, because of the pain in her arthritic joints while her four strong healthy daughters were rude about her in her presence. Vile, actually, at times. Memories of occasions when she was so drunk that she *forgot who we were*. And there are memories which even now, seven years after her death, are too precious or too painful for public processing.

When she died I was due to see her only three weeks later. She had rung me a few weeks before, and she was lonely and sad. Her only great friend left in the village had died horribly of cirrhosis a few months before— obviously a danger of English village life. She missed him terribly, as well, perhaps, as sensing the path down which she must inevitably travel, even while continuing to pretend that all was well with the world. We talked and she even cried a bit on the phone, and I told her that I would see her soon, but sadly it wasn't soon enough.

Thankfully she had been out here only the year before, and it was so obvious then that this was the last time she would be able to make the trip, we had, I felt, really made the best of it, given by then her almost constantly tipsy state. But for a long time I felt as if she could have at least waited to die until I had got to England to visit her!

When she died I was sitting on our verandah at the coast, prior to driving back to Sydney for a dinner party. I didn't know then that was the time, but I was, as it transpired, thinking of her a lot during her final hours. Somehow that thought has always comforted me.

Sam is a Pisces, like Julia, and he talks about her a lot. He knows she broke her neck, he knows she loved drawing. He loves the wildflower paintings of hers that we have at our beach house, and he asks me unanswerable child questions like: 'What happened to Julia's blood, Mummy, did it just dry up like a rusty old nail?' I try and answer him as honestly as I can. I tell him what I do truly believe, that this life is merely a part of something much bigger, and although we cannot see Julia, she is still around us, and part of us in very many ways. He doesn't know yet that she was an alcoholic—maybe he never will, maybe he will. I don't know. It is part of my story I think, not part of his. In the meantime I continue the journey of my relationship with my mother through my child, and I find that a great blessing.

ANNE KIRKPATRICK
Travelling Another Road

As the car pulled away, I could still remember my confusion at suddenly re-entering that 'other world'—the one before my daughter Kate was born. I'd lost all track of time after the birth and couldn't have cared less if World War III had started. The world outside the hospital just ceased to exist. I was happy beyond words with my little baby daughter and nothing else mattered.

The actual birth was over after only four hours at the hospital, since, living only five minutes away, I'd stayed home as long as I could. I was happy with my hospital birth experience, since there were no major complications and luckily I was able to get by without any drugs, which was the way

I'd wanted it. I don't remember consciously being in control throughout the birth, but rather being within myself, surrendering to the waves of contractions overwhelming my body, willing my baby to be born, and steadfastly believing in my body's ability to do it. And then that moment when all was still after the storm of contractions was like no other moment I've ever experienced.

I'd never imagined myself as particularly maternal, was never one to want my turn to nurse and gurgle over someone else's baby. But all that changed the moment Kate was placed on my tummy. I was a goner, a convert for life. To experience that moment a second time around when my son James was born was all the sweeter.

I remember the tremendous relief I felt afterwards, flopped on a chair under the shower, feeling totally wasted, looking at my funny, slack stomach, and feeling so at peace and happy that Kate and I had both come through the birth OK, as had millions of other women and babies the world over. This had been my consoling thought since that time in my pregnancy when I'd realised this was a one-way street and I'd become a bit nervous about the birth.

Now, three months later, Kate and I were heading off on a five-week tour of Queensland with the Slim Dusty Show, and as the car pulled away from our flat in Crows Nest, I felt torn.

'Why don't you come on the Queensland tour with us? It'll help get your hand back in and we'll help with Kate,' Mum and Dad had said.

After all, they had hit the road with me in tow when I was two—in a caravan, camping behind local halls and making do, often with no washing machine available. Now we would be staying in motels with all facilities— LUXURY!

But it seemed I'd travelled somewhere else that last 12 months and I wasn't sure if I was ready, or even wanted to go back. I'd loved being pregnant—it slowed me down and gave me time out from my restlessness to enjoy each moment, happy to let my body follow its natural course. I was leaving behind my husband who I knew missed Kate so, and found it hard to understand why I needed to head off on tour so soon after the birth.

But that restless part of me was calling again. In this game, the longer you're out of it, the harder it is to come back, and the 'greener' your voice and stage manner. So, on the other hand, I was glad of the chance to start work again and, in family tradition, it seemed quite natural to take Kate along with me. I can't say my decision hasn't caused both Greg and I some heartache over the years, but we just seem to keep working through it.

We survived that first tour. Mum and Dad were very sweet, organising my meals as I travelled, breastfed, crashed out for a nap while Kate slept, sang, breastfed, travelled, napped, sang... Three weeks into the tour I was on stage in Bundaberg and I could hear between verses the sounds of Kate's wails wafting in from outside the hall where Mum was frantically wheeling her up and down in the hope of lulling her off to sleep. We all three were wondering whatever made us think that Kate at three months would just slot into our touring schedule.

It also upset her feeding pattern and I went through a nightmarish week of sore, swollen breasts when Kate wouldn't feed. I desperately tried bottles with my expressed milk—everything and anything until she finally settled down again.

After that first bumpy tour, though, Kate and I were on and off the road for the next three years, and my life since then has been one big juggling act.

By the time I fell pregnant with my son James, my career was cruising along nicely. I even took my husband by surprise with my timing—my body and I had just decided that the time was right, after only a half-hearted effort on my part at keeping up the rhythm method.

But no one was more surprised than Doug Ashdown's manager. Doug and I had been doing a lot of shows together, dueting and also working up demos of songs with a view to recording an album together and subsequent touring to promote it. There were big plans afoot. I had all this fabulous gear that had been made especially for me during the filming of the *Slim Dusty Movie*—a turquoise suede outfit with red hand-stitching, a silver and mauve suede dress, and a white leather dress with diamantés and fringes. I was going through my Rhinestone Cowgirl phase!

I just didn't have the heart to tell them all immediately, but one night when I knew that I couldn't squeeze into the white leather dress any longer, I broke the news.

So, the duet album with Doug never came to pass. I was sorry about that as Doug's voice and mine blended beautifully and it would have been a great album.

Well, I had people telling me that my timing was lousy and that my career would go down the tube, but James wouldn't have been my delightful sunshiny little boy without that timing. Anyway, my most successful album, *Out of the Blue*, and the subsequent highest profile time of my career, didn't happen until much later, in 1990, which says a lot for so-called 'timing'.

The trouble was, I'd also taken a lot of advance bookings, so the year I was pregnant with James was full of surprises. Like the time I hopped off the plane at Port Pirie in South Australia for its annual Country Music Festival. I could tell just by the looks on the faces of the people waiting that they hadn't expected their star attraction to turn up six months pregnant.

Even though I'd appeared at the Gympie Muster Festival only a month before and managed fine, it was a month extra into a second pregnancy, which can make a big difference. I was huge, and feeling it. I sort of stood out among the wide-eyed svelte young things who were gathered in groups backstage, all excited at their oncoming performances. I hung back in the dressing room with my feet up until the very last second before I had to go on stage, wondering where on earth I was going to summon the energy from to get through an hour-and-a-quarter bracket. But, in true tradition, the show must go on—and even though I'm sure I looked very much like a toffee apple on a stick in my green jersey pantsuit, somehow I got through the performance.

I was very relieved that I hadn't taken any other bookings up until James's birth.

Again, I was four hours in the hospital before James was born, and again I was very withdrawn, muttering and concentrating hard, which must have been frustrating for Greg who was with me throughout—as he had been with Kate—supporting and encouraging me. The bossy sister looking after me who was monitoring the heartbeat (and who insisted I was having a girl), was getting a bit edgy when the doctor still hadn't fronted and James's shoulders were wedged, stopping any further progress. As I puffed gallantly, becoming more bug-eyed and panicky by the second, the doctor's partner appeared (it just so happened that the one I'd seen for the last nine months had his day off—don't you just hate that!) and quickly reached in, turned James's shoulders, and my little boy was born.

I breastfed James for nine months, as I had with Kate, and when I took a gig in Barmera, South Australia, James was six months old and so I just took him along. But as

Greg saw me off at the airport, with James under one arm, and loaded up with guitar, disposable nappies, stroller, stage gear and the rest, he reckoned he definitely had the best deal staying home to take care of Kate.

From then on my career started accelerating again. Since I'd made the decision to do that first five-week tour with Kate, I'd kept my career going, no matter what. The phone would ring and I'd be saying, 'Yes, sure, I can do that date, it sounds great'. I'd put the phone down and say to myself, 'Anne, you've done it again. How can you possibly do that date? Greg's working, what'll you do with the kids, *and* it's an overnighter ...' And I'd start the frantic round of calls to organise a band, rehearsals, and my own preparation. Every gig for a while there was like putting together a jigsaw puzzle, and without my family network—my in-laws, my parents when they could, and Greg, all babysitting for me—I'd never have got through. I'm eternally grateful to them all.

At the same time, I was totally involved in those wonderful preschool years with my children. I wanted to give them all the experiences I could, take them places, show them things, play with them, read to them. I'd spend hours cooking and decorating birthday cakes, making playdough, and doing all those little things that are so rewarding. But I was starting to feel the strain of holding both worlds together.

James, like most babies, had an interesting sleeping pattern, to say the least. At the time, we were living in one of four flats in an old block that had a wonderful common backyard with a huge jacaranda tree. I spent many bleary-eyed mornings in that backyard, comparing notes on how much sleep I'd got with Michelle and Ann from downstairs who had children of a similar age. I know there are methods and books written on the subject of getting your baby to sleep right through the night, but the reality is that you just manage the best you can, and most new mothers exist in a zombie-like state for about the first 12 months of their babies' lives.

Even so, my first panic attack came out of the blue. I was travelling up to the Blue Mountains for some time off with my family after recently spending an anxious week in the Sydney Eye Hospital with James (who'd been stung in the eye by some beastie in our garden) when it hit.

My body just seemed to spiral out of control. I thought I was going to have a heart attack, or at worst die! My heart was racing and pounding, my breath came in quick, shallow gasps, and all I could do was sit on the ground with my legs clasped to me in an almost foetal position, and hope for it to pass—which it did after some minutes. It left me exhausted and frightened. I'd never heard of panic/anxiety attacks, but after seeking help, discovered I was not alone. I learned some specific breathing and relaxation exercises, but, more importantly, I learned to recognise the warning signals and respond. I only suffered a few more attacks before they disappeared completely.

My career took off, I recorded *Out of the Blue*, the kids

had started school, and even though our house looked like a nuclear waste zone sometimes, the 'juggling' seemed to be getting easier.

'But she's perceived as the mother of two children'— SHOCK, HORROR!—a record executive said recently while discussing my career. Yes, I'm a mother, a singer, a wife, and the best bloody juggler of the three you're ever likely to come across, and as I travel down this ever-unfolding road I wouldn't have it any other way.

When I agreed to contribute this piece I saw it as a wonderful indulgence to be able to write about my thoughts on the subject. It made me remember those moments, sometimes gut-wrenching, that catch you unawares as you feel your children's growing pains. The desire to make everything right for them. The soaring love you feel when you see them feeling good about themselves, happy with an achievement of their own. A look in my 15-year-old daughter's eyes, intense, quizzical, slightly worried, that takes me back to a moment soon after her birth when I looked into her huge eyes and first 'knew' her. A bellylaugh from my 11-year-old son that makes me want to ruffle his hair and hug him until he finally yells, 'Stop, Mum, far out!' in exasperation. That love, its ebb and flow, always sustaining, never drying up.

All these moments and so many more make me content to travel down this road.

CHRISTINE ANU
Kuiam

I grew up in a family of five children, and that is a small one compared to your average black family. The extended family is a part of life in our indigenous community.

Our 'small' family, consisting of Mum, Dad, myself, three other sisters and our only brother, resided in a three-bedroom house called Louisiana. In this house we lived with two of Dad's unmarried sisters and between them a tribe of 11 of our cousins.

Everyday chores would vary from emptying the thunder box and filling large 44-gallon drums with separate water for drinking and washing from the fresh-water spring well about a hundred metres or so from Louisiana, to changing many a miserable bum, keeping young ones entertained or making sure no one drowned in our front yard, which was the beach.

I suppose I started thinking about never having children of my own at this impressionable stage of my life. And I suppose when I voiced my thoughts I was told that all young girls say the same thing. But I was adamant that I was not going to wind up with the biggest unpaying job. Besides, a lot of young girls my age were falling pregnant and leaving school. I was determined not to follow suit by avoiding having babies altogether, at any time.

My observations were that the mother never really received any help unless there were older children. My mother was a dedicated mother and housewife and that was the only job she ever had. She gave all us children her full love and attention, and we'd do anything she'd ask, most of the time. My sister Helen and I are the oldest and a year apart and we were mostly in charge of looking after the younger children.

Bathing, changing nappies, dressing, feeding and entertaining. We pretty much accepted this as a part of growing up. After all Mum couldn't do everything, although we sometimes expected her to. 'I've only got two arms!'; 'You've got eyes, why don't you go find them?'; 'I've said "no" a thousand times, what part couldn't you understand?'. I can hear my mother saying these things like it was yesterday. I wonder if that will be me harping on to my son in a few years from now. I smile at the thought. Probably!

I remember how hard it was for my mother because

custom is that the daughter-in-law, or in this case sister-in-law, takes over running the household. She ran a big busy household without the help of running water, electricity, or even an electric generator. This house was just a shelter, it was so far beyond repair or maintenance. You could see underneath the house through the floorboards. The roof leaked all over and there were no ceilings. Any time of day you could spot large rats making their way around the roof beams towards their nests, which were amidst large trunks of clothing.

At an early age I'd already worked out how I could substitute pregnancy—adoption! But traditional adoption, without the headache of paperwork and the involvement of non-family members. Having children myself was totally out of the question. Seeing Mum with her workload only reiterated that thought. Culturally and traditionally, adopting out, or more appropriately 'giving', a child meant that the child would be brought up amongst family. Customarily your firstborn was given to your parents, or any other child to childless relatives, or just as a gift to a relative's family, thus extending the family. Ronald is the last one in our family and the only boy. He was 'given' to us by traditional adoption. My brother knows he was adopted but most traditionally adopted children are unaware or find out later in life. I was nine when Ronald arrived. He was the reason why helping Mum out was so delightful but, boy, was he spoilt rotten! Having Ronald with us really taught me how not to do things.

They say that parents don't get a degree in how to raise their children, but children will be parents too one day and we all manage the best we know how. In observing my parents I believe that their room for error was so that I could try something different if I decided to go down their path.

I graduated from school in 1987, an experience I felt that I didn't want to revisit in this lifetime. In hindsight, however, no matter how boring or inappropriate I felt school was, I know it provides many skills that we need to carry with us in life. But as institutionalised as the education system is, and with all its positive changes and improvements, no amount of schooling had taught me the skill of patience. Patience I would only find when I became a mother myself!

Another inevitable encounter in life other than school, and something I discovered while I was at school, was sex. Unfortunately, you couldn't have sex without the possibility of falling pregnant. I had to find out the hard way while I was studying at dance college. I fell pregnant to my now boyfriend of eight years when we'd only been seeing each other for six months. One of the hardest decisions in my life was not to go through with the pregnancy—there were so many reasons why I should and shouldn't. I soon learned that, as alone as I was left to make such a decision, the whole world seemed to have an opinion either directly or indirectly. Abortion is still such a taboo subject that when a woman decides against proceeding with the pregnancy there seems to be little or no support. My friends and family supported my decision but, as I found out, not the act itself. I realised that couples need support whether they decide to have a family or not. But I knew, too, that when the time came when I decided to become a parent, it would be the most perfectly right thing at the right time, and that it would be the most unforgettable experience!

Come 1995 and big things seem to be waiting for my arrival. I'm anxious because I can sense something brewing, and I'm powering on, a generator of nervous energy. I can't eat or sleep any more and my appetite for love and sex grows insatiable. My life, however, still seems to dwell around the 'I'm due for my period and it still hasn't come' factor.

I was on the return flight from the Asian tour of my debut album and quite an emotional bundle. I was looking forward to landing at Sydney airport and running over to the departure lounge to meet up with my boyfriend who was leaving for Vanuatu. I couldn't wait to see him and tell him how much the world pissed me off yesterday, today and not to mention right now. Then after all that I'd tell him how I'd missed him. Albert listened for a few seconds then asked me if I'd had my period at all. I saw Albert off then went home myself feeling quite annoyed about what he'd asked, because I really couldn't remember!

The first time ever that I'm not worried about my next period and I'm having a nice fuzzy dream. I dream that I can see a little coffee-coloured bubba sitting amongst my soft toy collection above my wardrobe and the baby is smiling at me. I smile back at the baby and he says, 'I'm a little boy and I'm with you'. I shudder in my sleep and lose the vision and wake up.

I woke up realising I needed to confirm if I was pregnant or not! DUH!

When I was more interested in stuffing sushi, sashimi, a McFeast and junior burger, large fries and a large Sprite down past my tired vocal cords into an eagerly awaiting stomach, I wasn't shocked out of my brains to learn I was preggers. Suddenly the fears of looking like a queen-sized mattress for ever and ever just vanished. I'd had so many fears because I was concerned about my outward appearance. Fears like looking fat and never being thin again, having a weak bladder or a failed sex life, because no one could just pop back into place after being stretched 'down there' beyond one's physical limits! My understanding had always been that pregnancy and giving birth was a major physical and psychological feat that rightfully no one should be able to survive. But they do! Being pregnant, I came to understand how simple and beautiful life really is. Having children is a blessing and being the guardian of another little life should bring many a valuable lesson. I look forward to my life!

I worked for the entire pregnancy. I was thankful to be

able to work at my own pace and be surrounded by support, but I hated being treated like an invalid in some cases, as pregnancy is a normal fact of life. One aspect of my pregnancy was that it didn't seem to affect how much work I received. In fact, work seemed to increase! However, I was working through a pregnancy with nine months (or was it more like 12?) of relentless 24-hour a day gagging or dry retching. Intimate moments face to face with my breakfast/lunch/dinner. But I needed all that work, I felt, as a psychological meter that would help me through my home birth—a decision that was becoming scarier as I came to the realisation that Albert was just not going to be a support person. As much as we wanted it his work commitments didn't allow it. However, working made me feel normal and most of the time I was treated like everyone else. After a while my stomach became invisible. It just wasn't an issue.

It would be a home birth because I didn't want too much interference or distraction. Giving birth was not going to be treated as a hospital formality. This was going to be the most important gig of my entire young life because I felt I would have a lot to offer my child. The people I chose to be present at my labour were my sister Helen and a friend who just happened to be a traditional lay midwife, Barbara. The room for the birth, the 'special' room as I termed it, hadn't been decided upon as yet. I felt it was something that would work itself out. Along with enough plastic to cover every bit of furniture with a bit left over for the floors, walls and ceilings! Besides, the hospital was five minutes up the road and my GP and obstetrician were on call should any difficulties arise. I anticipated no difficulties, that it would be only as difficult as I wanted to make it. I wanted my home birth to be a pleasant, memorable experience for all involved. There were the familiar surroundings. I thought, How could I go wrong? And I wouldn't have to spend a cent. I looked after my health and fitness better than I ever had. There was not one decision I'd made that I was doubtful about and I wasn't about to be scared out of this choice and these decisions. I was all so ready, thinking, Okay, where are you baby? Weeks passed and then two months, and then I was a whopping 37-and-a-half weeks (supposedly), of pregnant woman whose waters had just ruptured.

After two days I'd diagnosed myself as having the piddles out of control until the urge to have a bowel movement wouldn't go away and I still had the piddles. I thought to be on the safe side I should call Albert in Melbourne and tell him to begin his hike up to Sydney. Next on the list was Helen and then Barbara and then my management. I gave Helen a list of people's names to cancel appointments though my management had done this as soon as they were notified that I'd gone into labour. Even though I didn't lose my cool once through the labour, I was quite annoyed that no one else around me was panicking or kicking up a fuss. I mean, Get with the program guys! I'm having a @*#*ing baby!

Let's see. My waters broke on the Wednesday and labour started at three am on Friday—I think I slept through most of it. True labour was 15 minutes! Hey! I'm proud of that! I'm also proud of how I learned to love and respect my body from the inside as a result of having a little person grow inside me.

Albert and I always wanted to name our son Kuiam. In Torres Strait legend Kuiam was a feared head-hunter. His mother was Torres Strait Islander and his father's origins were from the Cape York area. The fact that Kuiam's background combined both indigenous cultures was the main reason for going with that name.

I believe our parents gave us names in English that were deliberately easy to pronounce, thinking that it would save a lot of trouble and bother with pronunciation and meaning, but not realising they were assisting in slowly eliminating our language—the core of culture. We need to keep our language alive, at least in our families in one form or another. It's great fun teaching people to say 'Kuiam', because mostly people find it difficult to pronounce. And at least my son will have an interesting story to tell about the origins of his name.

I met my son Kuiam Eliotha Yunggulama Gunumbalwuy Galaku Anu-David at 12:30 pm on Friday 17 May 1996. Albert stumbled up the stairs four minutes into the event, fumbled around a bit before managing a sure grip on the clamps, and disconnected our son from inside me forever. Then he appeared to be in shock. I think it was a combination of snipping the umbilical cord and having a six-pound, three-ounce life in front of him that made him a little speechless for days. But Albert did a lot and was willing to do more if you showed him how. My mother came and stayed while Albert was away and she was a tremendous help and support and gave me a lot of information during and after the birth about traditional customs relating to childbirth and child rearing. She encouraged me with handling such a tiny person, and her presence helped me through post-natal depression, which I suspect every woman suffers from to certain degrees.

A lot of family secrets started to surface whenever I would have conversations with my mother. I feel my relationship with her has opened up since I became a mother myself. It's like I am now an initiated woman after experiencing the pain of childbirth. This observation with my mother reminded me of how pregnancy and motherhood is viewed by a lot of women in our culture, especially regarding younger women. A couple of times I heard one particular comment from different women relatives regarding my pregnant belly: 'Oh! you proper nice gal, and you go and you spoil yourself them kind!'; and it never really made sense to me—except that customarily the thinking was that life ended when you chose to start a family. Perhaps what was being frowned upon were the missed opportunities.

To this extent I hope that the choice I've made to be a mother and a career woman is a positive example to young Torres Strait women—that a career is also a child that is growing and in need of nurturing, and that there is also room for nurturing a career in parenthood.

Notes on Contributors

Christine Anu is a singer, dancer, actor and songwriter. Born in Cairns, of Torres Strait Islander descent, she has performed as a dancer both in Australia and overseas with the Bangarra Dance Theatre. Christine's 1995 album *Stylin' Up* reached gold status and in 1996 she was awarded an ARIA award for Best Female Performer and Best Indigenous Artist. She currently lives in Sydney.

Candida Baker was born in London in 1955, and emigrated to Australia in 1977, where she is now a citizen. Her first novel, *Women and Horses*, was published in 1990; her second book of fiction is *The Powerful Owl*, a collection of stories. She is also the creator of the well-known series

Yacker: Australian Writers Talk about their Work. As a journalist she has worked on the *Age*, *Time Australia*, the *Times on Sunday*, and the *Good Weekend* magazine, and she is currently Arts Editor of the *Sydney Morning Herald*.

Penny Biggins is a performer, musician and writer. She lives in Sydney with her husband and son.

Jane Cadzow is a journalist who writes for the *Good Weekend*, the Saturday magazine of the *Sydney Morning Herald* and the *Age*. She has one son and lives in Canberra.

Kerry Cue is a humourist who taught maths and science for 10 diabolical years, gave birth, discovered humour and wrote books, including her latest, *Australia Unbuttoned*. She lives in the Melbourne suburb of Ivanhoe with her husband, two children, a budgerigar, a guinea pig and an ailing fish tank.

Ursula Dubosarsky is a children's novelist whose books include *The White Guinea Pig*, which won both the Victorian and NSW state awards for children's literature in 1994, and *The First Book of Samuel*, which won the NSW Ethnic Affairs Commision award in 1995, and was named an Honour Book by the Children's Book Council of Australia in 1996. Her latest books are *Bruno and the Crumhorn* and *Black Sails, White Sails*. She lives in Sydney with husband Avi, daughter Maisie, son Dover and baby Bruno.

Fiona Giles is a writer and academic presently living in New York City with her husband and son. She is the editor of *Dick for a Day* (Random House, forthcoming 1997).

Trisha Goddard has worked as a journalist, television presenter and producer, spending (amongst many other things) over two years as the NSW presenter of the ABC's *7.30 Report*, and the last nine years as a member of the *Play School* team. She is the producer of health and lifestyle programs and videos and is especially committed to issues concerning mental health. She is a single mother with two daughters, Billie, aged seven, and Madison, aged two.

Sue Ingleton is an actor and director who began performing her own work in the mid-1970s. She has also written and directed for Circus Oz, Gerry Connolly and Sue Ann Post, and is well-known in theatre and television, last appearing in *Mercury* for ABC TV. Her publications include *Sue Ingleton's Almaniac*, and stories in *Ink: The Follow Me Short Story Winners* and *Weddings and Wives* (ed Dale Spender). She also teaches drama and creative writing, and runs workshops in energy alignments and sacred theatre.

Susan Johnson was born in 1956 and worked as a journalist before taking up fiction writing full time. She is the author of four novels, most recently *Hungry Ghosts* (Pan Macmillan 1996) and is the editor of the Random House anthology *Women Love Sex* (1996). After six years in Paris, Hong Kong and London, she returned to Australia in 1995 and currently lives in Melbourne with her second husband and their son. She is expecting a second child in 1997. 'This Is My Life' is an extract from a work-in-progress about the experience of motherhood.

Karina Kelly graduated from Sydney University with an arts degree in 1980. She has worked in television for 16 years, first in news at SBS and Sydney's Channel Seven, and then for the ABC TV science program *Quantum*. She is the narrator of the children's TV program *Bananas in Pyjamas*, and is a member of the boards of the Near Eastern Archaeology Foundation of Sydney University and the Council of the National Museum of Australia. She is married with a son, Adam.

Gretel Killeen has written and performed comedy for stage, radio and television for the past 10 years. She is the author of seven books, the single mother of two children, the voice behind innumerable radio and television commercials, and completely and utterly exhausted.

Anne Kirkpatrick, singer, is the daughter of Slim Dusty and Joy McKean. She spent her early childhood on the road with the Slim Dusty Show, and later followed this tradition by touring with her own children. Her last album, *Anne Kirkpatrick and Friends—Live*, celebrated 21 years of solo recording. Of her nine albums, her most successful has been *Out of the Blue*, released in 1991, for which she won an ARIA award as well as two Golden Guitars at the Tamworth Country Music Awards. Anne is an active member of the Country Music Association of Australia. She now lives in Sydney with her husband, Greg, and two children, Kate and James, and is currently working on songs for a new album.

Donna McDonald is a former social worker and government policy advisor, who now manages a Brisbane theatre company, La Boite Theatre. Her first book, *Jack's Story* (1991), recounted her journey from new motherhood upon the birth and subsequent death, five-and-a-half months later, of her son Jack.

Sally McInerney has five children aged 25, 23, 22 and 10 (times two), and is completing a book called *Leaving the Island*, a home-grown ethnographic story of childhood and little children.

Debra Oswald has written for stage, television and film, and has had two children's books published. Her plays include *Dags* and *Gary's House* and her television credits include *Police Rescue*, *Palace of Dreams*, *Sweet and Sour* and *Bananas in Pyjamas*. She lives in Sydney and has two sons.

Rosie Scott is a writer whose books include *Glory Days*, *Queen of Love*, *Nights with Grace*, *Feral City*, *Lives on Fire* and *Movie Dreams*. She has two children and lives in Sydney.

Margaret Simons, 36, was for 10 years a reporter on the *Age*, winning a High Commendation in the 1990 Walkley Awards for her stories on the Victorian police, before resigning in 1991 to write her first novel, *The Ruthless*

Garden, which won the inaugural Angus & Robertson Bookworld prize in 1993. Since then she has divided her time between freelance journalism, mainly for the *Australian*, and her own writing. Her first daughter, Clare, was born in May 1996, and her second novel, *The Truth Teller*, was published in June 1996.

Jill Singer until recently was the Victorian presenter of Channel Seven's current affairs program, *Today Tonight*. She has also worked for the Channel Ten network and for the ABC, where she spent 10 years in radio and television, reporting as well as developing and producing programs; she also spent several years working on the *7.30 Report*. She has won a number of awards for journalism, including a Walkley Award for Best Television Investigative Journalist in 1992. She has a science degree, no husband, two dogs, one daughter, and a lust for trouble.

Debbie Spillane is a sports writer as well as a television and radio presenter. She was sideline reporter on ABC TV rugby league telecasts and a regular on the sports comedy program *Live & Sweaty*. For three years she was co-host of Triple J's drivetime program *Hard Coffee*. She has two daughters, Jemima and Eleanor, and lives in Sydney.

Leonie Stevens was born during the Cuban missile crisis, and grew up in Melbourne. She is the author of *Nature Strip* and *Big Man's Barbie*, and the editor of *Pub Fiction*, a collection of site-specific stories by cool new writers. Her stories have appeared in anthologies and magazines, and on radio and the Net. She and her partner Paul have a seven-year-old daughter, Amaelia, who has a wicked sense of humour and her father's eyes. Leonie's next novel is *Glue*.

Jenny Tabakoff was born in Sydney in 1959, and trained as a journalist on the *Sydney Morning Herald*. After nine years working in London on the staff of the *Times* and the *Daily Telegraph*, she returned in 1995 to Australia and the *Herald*, where she is now a columnist and feature writer. She lives deep in Sydney suburbia with her husband and two sons, aged three and six.